Resistance Band Workout

A Simple Way to Tone and Strengthen Your Muscles

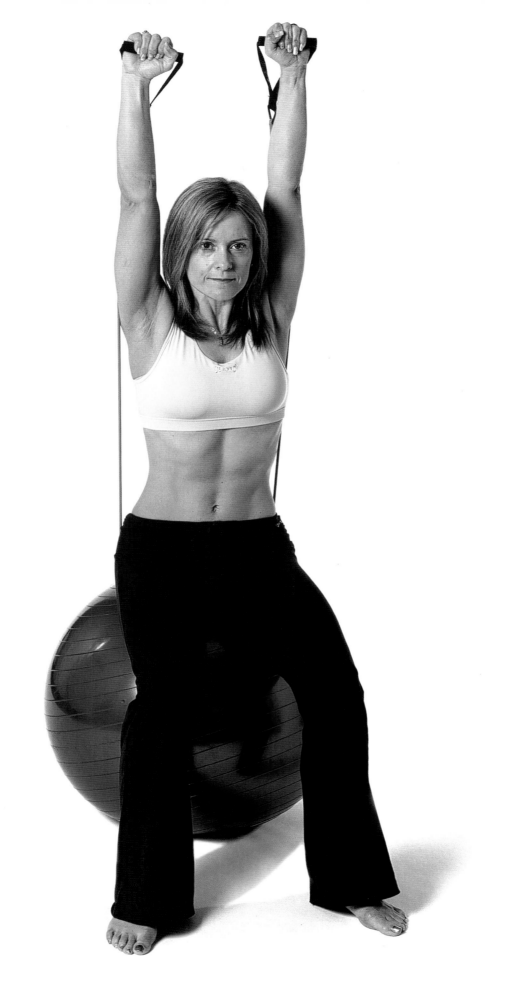

Resistance Band Workout

A Simple Way to Tone and Strengthen Your Muscles

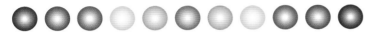

James Milligan

PRC

Produced 2004 by
PRC Publishing Limited
The Chrysalis Building
Bramley Road, London W10 6SP

An imprint of **Chrysalis** Books Group

This edition published 2004
Distributed in the U.S. and Canada by:
Sterling Publishing Co., Inc.
387 Park Avenue South
New York, NY 10016

ISBN 1-85648-724-5

Printed and bound in Malaysia

ACKNOWLEDGMENTS
The publisher wishes to thank Simon Clay for taking all the photography in this book,
including the photographs on the front and back covers. All photography is copyright © Chrysalis Images 2004.
Thanks also to Proactive-Health.co.uk for providing the exercise equipment used in the book.

SAFETY NOTE
The exercises are for information only and are not intended to replace appropriate advice from a qualified practitioner.
Any person suffering from conditions requiring medical attention should consult a qualified medical practitioner
before undertaking any exercises from this book.

Contents

Introduction

Theory Behind Resistance Band Training

The term resistance training refers to using an increased force against a body movement for the purpose of developing greater muscle tone, strength, endurance, and power. Resistance training can also provide other benefits such as improved weight control through increased metabolism, as well as injury prevention. In recent years resistance training has become an integral part of a balanced fitness routine. Traditionally, to include this type of training into your lifestyle would mean joining a gym or investing in large and heavy exercise equipment. Not everybody has the luxury of a gym membership or the space to install home equipment, but there is a way to get all the benefits of resistance training without either of these things.

The solution is the resistance band. Made from pliable materials such as rubber and latex, resistance bands are compact, light, and safe. These bands were first used in physical rehabilitation to aid recovery from injury and illness. Now they are widely used in aerobic studies and homes around the world.

Benefits of Using Resistance Bands

Low cost

Resistance bands provide training without the use of expensive equipment or the need to join a gym. For the price of one month's gym membership, or less, you can set yourself up with everything you need for a complete resistance workout.

Lightweight

Unlike other resistance training equipment that provides resistance through weight, the bands are light, making them easier and safer to move around.

Storage and portability

Because the bands are lightweight and compact they do not require any storage space, unlike bulky free weights and benches. This also means that you can take them anywhere, which is especially beneficial when traveling, enabling you to maintain exercise consistency.

Constant resistance during exercise movement

Resistance training equipment normally provides gravity-generated resistance, which means it can be lost during some parts of the exercise. Bands provide constant resistance throughout the exercise, and therefore more benefit.

Time efficiency

You can plan your time more efficiently by using resistance bands, as you won't need to work around gym schedules or allow for additional traveling time. You can pick them up whenever you want and wherever you are.

Safe

The band only provides resistance when you want it. The resistance is progressive and controlled by you, making it safer and easier on the joints. This also makes it suitable for people of all ages. The bands eliminate the mishaps normally associated with resistance training, such as the risk of dropping heavy weights. Even with the improved safety, you should always consult a physician/doctor before beginning any kind of resistance training program.

What results can you expect from using resistance bands?

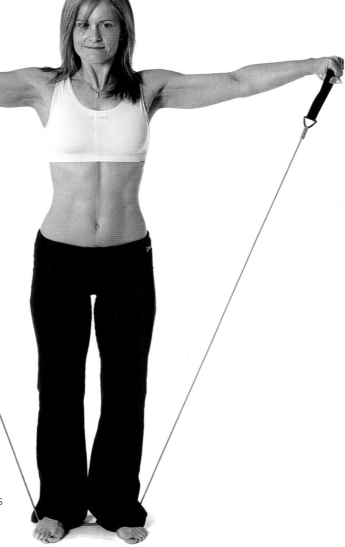

- Enhanced muscle tone, strength, endurance, power, and flexibility.
- Improved posture and support around joints.
- Greater flexibility and range of movement in joints.
- Improved metabolism, body weight control, and energy.
- Greater enjoyment of sports like golf, skiing, and tennis.
- Prevention of muscle and joint atrophy (loss of muscle mass) caused by aging.
- Improved bone protection and reduced risk of osteoporosis.
- Reduced risk of injury.

The terminology of the anatomy and muscle groups being worked in each section has been kept to a level where it is easily understandable for a beginner, yet is still informative to those who have a good basic knowledge of other training methods. It is outside the remit of this book to go into too much anatomical detail.

Safety Precautions

Before commencing any exercise with resistance bands, please check the following:

Ensure all equipment is in good working order:

- Examine the resistance band before each use, checking for small tears or punctures. Damage to the band can cause it to snap under tension. If you do find damage, discard it and replace it with a new one.

Band storage:

- Resistance bands should be stored at room temperature and in a dark place. Do not store the bands in sunlight, as long exposure may cause damage to the bands' elastic properties.

Exercise area:

- Give yourself plenty of free space to perform the exercises. Choose an area that is nonslip.

Correct and safe usage:

- Make sure that you understand how to do each exercise properly by carefully reading through and following the full instructions before starting your workout. Improper use may cause serious injury.
- When positioning the band around or attaching it to an anchor point, ensure that it is at the specified level for the exercise and is secure. Do not attach the band to any loose objects. If using a door, ensure that others around know this, and don't try to use the door.

- Do not use the resistance band in a way that may cause it to flick toward the head and cause facial injury.
- Select a band with a suitable level of intensity starting with the lowest. Only increase the level of resistance when you can comfortably complete the specified number of repetitions.
- Be careful not to place the band around any part of the body or limbs that could result in cutting off circulation.
- Work each muscle through a full range being careful not to hyperextend or lock the joint.
- Allow sufficient rest periods (48 hours) between resistance workouts for recovery and to prevent overtraining.
- If you are new to resistance training, it is advisable to build up the exercise intensity and frequency gradually. The 30 Minute Workout is an ideal place to start for the first four weeks. It is not advisable to start with one of the more advanced workouts such as the golf pogram.

Health:

- Some bands contain latex, which can cause an allergic reaction. There are latex-free bands available to prevent an adverse reaction.
- If you are new to exercise or have a medical condition, check with your doctor before commencing any form of exercise.

Equipment

For the exercises in this book you will require the following equipment:

Resistance bands: There are many types of band available. Traditionally the resistance band is without fixed handles. They are generally made of latex and come as a flat sheet (#2) in various thicknesses and colors, which denote the intensity of each band. A knot can be tied in each end to attach a handle or to make a loop to hold onto. The other type is generally referred to as a resistance tube (#1). These are mainly latex-free and come with handles already attached. Whichever you choose, be sure to get quality bands to limit the chance of them breaking. To avoid confusion, "bands" and "tubes" have been used in the same context within this book, and are called "bands".

Ankle strap: An ankle strap (#3) is required so that the band can be attached to it, and then comfortably placed around your leg for lower body exercises.

Door anchor: Some exercises require the band to be anchored to create a suitable resistance angle. The simple yet effective door anchor loop (#4) can be closed in the door to provide a solid anchor point. If there isn't a suitable doorway, the band can be placed around a pole or similar fixed object capable of holding that level of resistance.

Chair or swiss ball: Some exercises require a chair or similar object to sit or hold onto for balance.

How to choose the correct strength of band

Different manufacturers make bands of varied resistance levels in different colors. Be sure to follow their specific instructions. In this book we are using:

- Light resistance (yellow) is recommended for use by seniors, and to improve the smaller muscle groups of the upper body.
- Medium resistance (green) is for average strength, and to work small to medium muscle groups such as the back and hips.
- Heavy resistance (red) is recommended for the average man or active woman and can be used to develop muscle groups such as the arms, shoulders, chest, and legs.
- Extra heavy resistance (black) is recommended for use by advanced men and women to develop large and strong muscle groups.

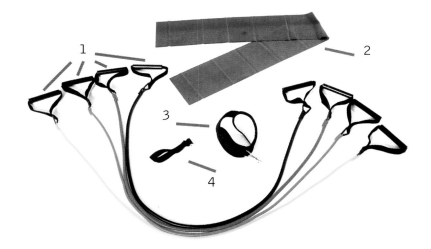

Muscle Areas

Muscle areas and names have been listed at the bottom of each exercise description throughout the book to give a better understanding of the areas that are being worked.

Major Anterior Muscle Groups

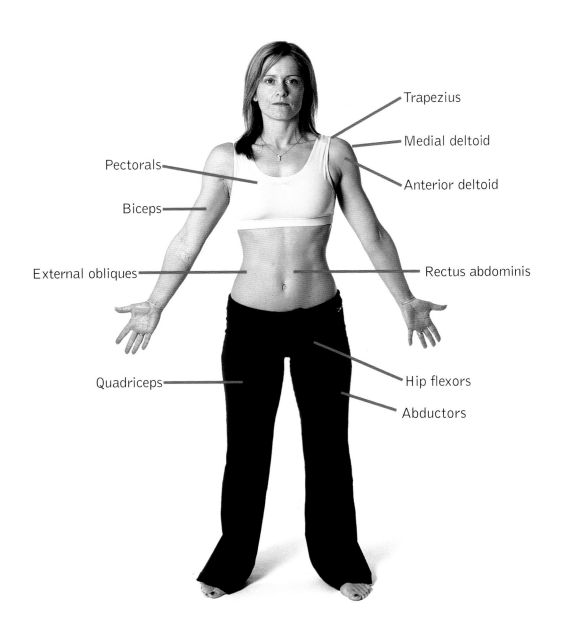

Trapezius

Medial deltoid

Pectorals

Anterior deltoid

Biceps

External obliques

Rectus abdominis

Quadriceps

Hip flexors

Abductors

Major Posterior Muscle Groups

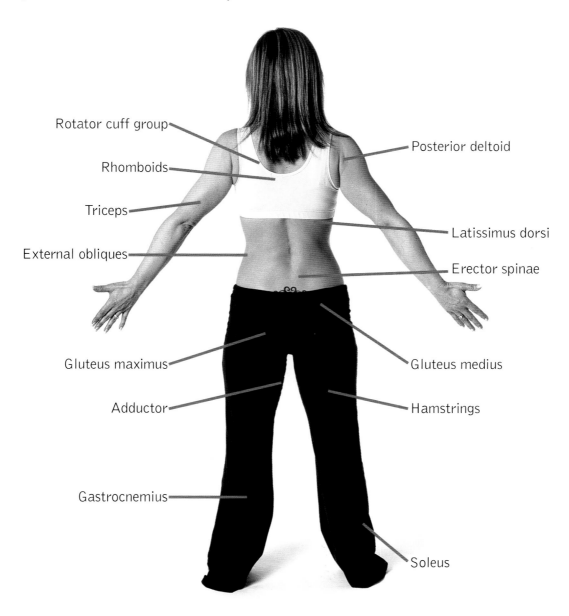

Rotator cuff group

Rhomboids

Triceps

External obliques

Gluteus maximus

Adductor

Gastrocnemius

Posterior deltoid

Latissimus dorsi

Erector spinae

Gluteus medius

Hamstrings

Soleus

Correct Exercise Posture

Correct postural positioning is imperative when exercising to prevent injury and to obtain the maximum benefit from your routine.

Poor posture:

Here is an example of poor posture. Many people unknowingly form this position with head down and shoulders rounded forward. This posture will only lead to problems in the future.

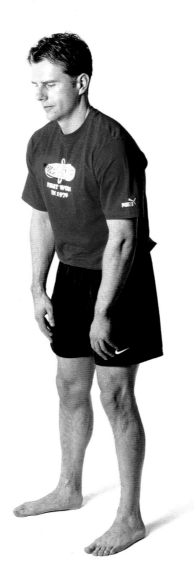

Correct posture:

Here is an example of good/correct posture.

- Standing tall, head and neck straight with eyes focused straight ahead.

- Shoulders relaxed and back, with chest out.

- Abdomen pulled in and muscles held tight.

- Pelvis curled under slightly so that buttocks are tucked in to form a neutral position.

- Feet placed hip width apart with weight distributed evenly and toes pointing forward.

- Knees slightly bent.

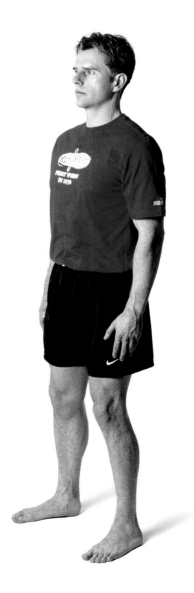

Grip Positions

Throughout the book, references will be made to the different grip positions required. They are as follows:

Overhand grip

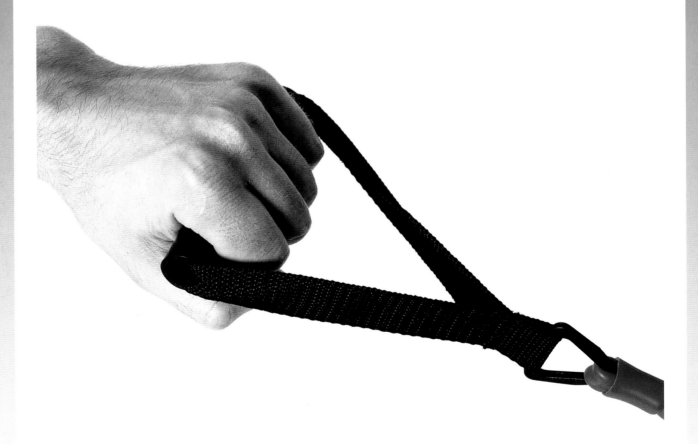

Underhand grip

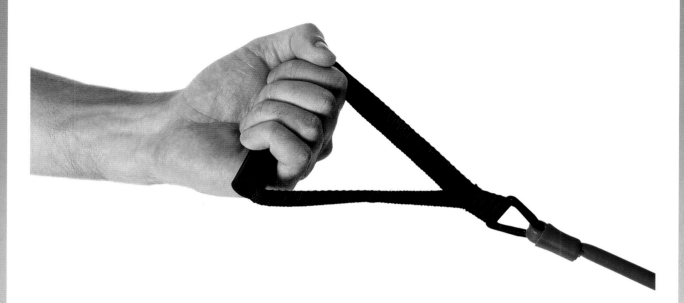

Palm-inward grip

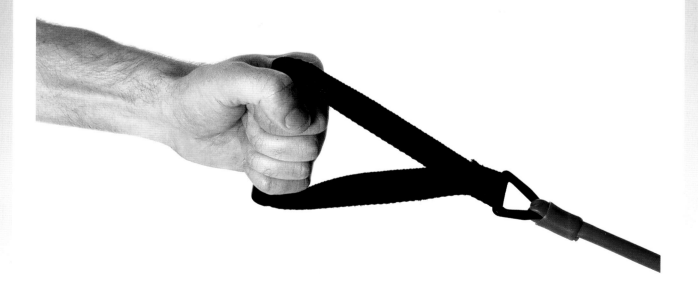

Warm Up

Warming up prior to strenuous exercise of any kind is crucial. Although it is often the part of the training program that many people miss out, this can be to the detriment of their workout.

Warming up before exercise with light aerobic and flexibility exercises is important because it:

- Prepares the muscles and joints for the activity ahead by increasing blood flow and muscle temperature.
- Reduces the risk of injury to muscles, tendons, and ligaments by making them more pliable, allowing movement through a full range of motions more safely and effectively.
- Encourages circulation to the muscles, heart, and lungs by raising the flow of blood. This increased blood volume helps supply muscles with additional oxygen and nutrients required for exercise.
- Increases central nervous system functions which help to enhance factors such as muscle control, psychology, and coordination. The improved frame of mind reduces the perception of effort when training with resistance bands, allowing more to be put into the workout.

A pre-resistance band warm-up should last at least 10 minutes and should focus on all areas of the body, no matter what exercises are about to be performed. This should start with light but brisk aerobic-style movements that work large muscle group areas together. This will increase blood flow and muscle temperature. Once this has been achieved, the muscles will be more pliable and ready for the flexibility phase of the warm up.

These exercises can also be used at the end of your workout as a cool-down phase, with very light aerobic movements to reduce heart rate. When performing resistance exercises your muscles tend to shorten with some of the fibers staying more contracted than normal. Performing flexibility exercises after the workout will help to correct and further improve muscle length, which will also aid recovery.

Here are some simple yet effective aerobic exercises that you can use in your pre-resistance band workout warm-up program in any environment:

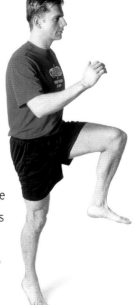

Jogging on the Spot
Gentle jogging is a great way of warming up as you are using the large muscle groups in your legs and controlling your body weight. You can do this on the spot, or moving forward as if in an open area.

To get the most from this exercise as a warm-up, progressively raise knees higher and use large opposite arm and leg movements, lifting hands to head level.

Star Jumps

Star jumps are good for warming up the areas that are not used much in jogging, because you are moving your limbs out to the side, rather than forward and backward in jogging. Therefore areas such as the middle of the shoulder, top of shoulder, outer thigh, and inner thigh are being prepared.

Start by standing straight with feet together and arms by your side. Jump feet out, landing in a wide stance and simultaneously lift arms out to the side and above your head, keeping them straight. As soon as your feet touch the floor, jump back to the start position and bring your arms back down. Continue to repeat this movement.

Shadow Punch / Leg Strides

This warm-up exercise is great as it allows you to progressively work the chest, arms, shoulders, and upper back, as well as legs, hips, and midsection through slight rotation. This also helps you to develop cross-body coordination by using an opposite arm and leg movement.

Start with one arm forward, the palm of your hand facing down, and in a fist, and the opposite leg forward. The other arm should be bent and close to your body with the palm of your hand facing up and a clenched fist, and opposite leg back. Keeping the weight on your toes, jump, swapping your leg position in one large stride. Simultaneously punch your other arm forward, bringing the extended one back. Once your toes have made contact with the ground, jump back to the start position and continue to repeat.

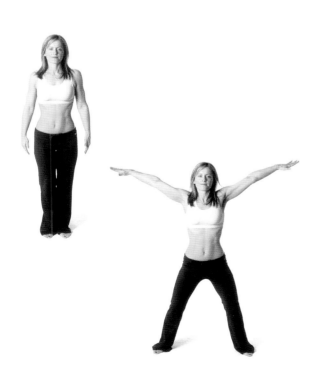

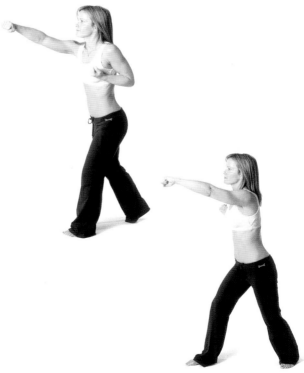

Flexibility Exercises

Back

Different things that we do each day, whether sitting or standing for long periods, bad posture, or stress, can all contribute to tension in the back. This is a great stretch to start with as it targets the whole length of the back.

Kneel down on the floor, sitting on your heels. Roll shoulders forward and curl your body over your thighs, tucking your head in with your arms relaxed by your side. Hold this position for 30 seconds, close your eyes and focus on relaxing each time you breathe out.

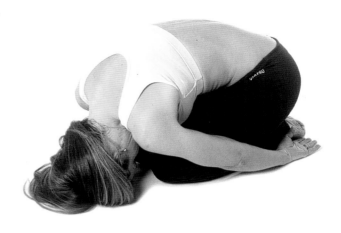

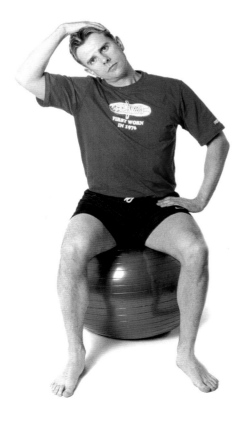

Neck Lateral Flexion

Many activities during the day cause tension in the upper shoulders and neck, especially if you are suffering from stress. The lateral neck stretch will help to release the tension and prevent further related problems.

Sit down so that your upper body is upright with your shoulders back and abdominal muscles tight to support your midsection. Make sure that you are not slouching. Lower your ear toward the shoulder of the same side, until you feel a stretch in the neck and shoulder of the opposite side. You can control and increase the stretch by placing your hand over your head and easing it a little further. Hold the stretch for 15 seconds and then repeat on the other side.

Neck Extension

Other areas of neck tension include the back and front of the neck. This stretch improves and corrects tension in the front of the neck. Position yourself sitting down as in the previous neck stretch. Ensure that you hold the correct posture with your upper body straight and shoulders back.

Raise your chin as high as possible, keeping your mouth closed. Hold this position for 15 seconds.

Neck Flexion

The neck flexion stretch follows on from the neck extension. This stretch improves and corrects tension in the back of the neck. Position yourself sitting down as in the previous neck stretch. Make sure that you hold the correct posture with your upper body straight and shoulders back.

Lower your chin toward your chest, keeping shoulders back and torso upright. Hold this position for 15 seconds.

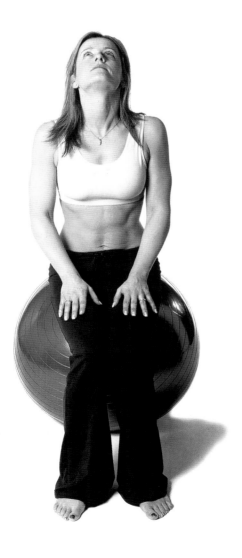

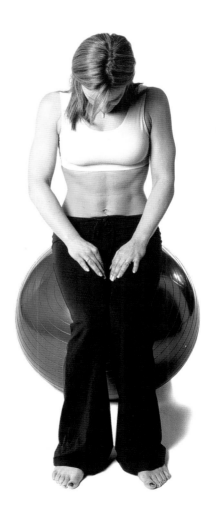

Lying Hamstrings

The hamstring group of muscles can become a problem area if a good level of flexibility is not maintained, causing other associated problems, especially in the lower back.

Start by lying flat on your back. Bend one leg at the knee, place the band over the foot of the other and extend it so that it is straight. Keeping your lower back and buttocks flat on the floor, flex the hip of the straight leg bringing your thigh back as far as possible without bending at the knee. Use the band to aid and progressively increase the stretch. Hold the stretch for 15 seconds and then repeat with the other leg.

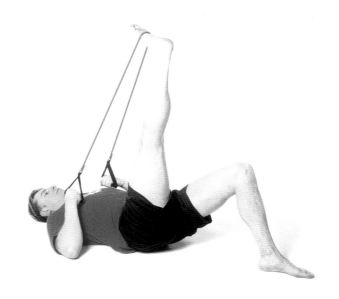

Seated Hamstrings and Torso Rotation

This is an additional hamstrings stretch which increases the range of the stretch in the upper position of the muscle group by adding a torso rotation.

Sit down on the floor with both legs straight. Sit tall with arms extended out to the side at shoulder height.

Rotate your torso aiming to get arms and shoulders parallel to your legs then lean forward reaching your hand to the outside of the opposite foot. Hold for 10 seconds then return back to the start position and repeat on the other side. Do this twice on each side. Make sure that your legs remain straight throughout the stretch and your buttocks stay flat on the floor.

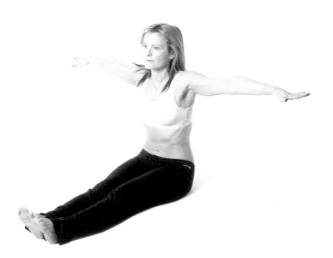
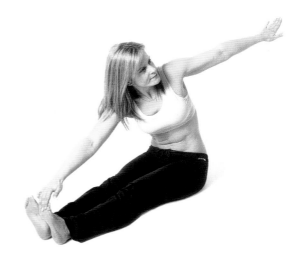

Gluteus—Knee to Chest

The gluteus group of muscles are located in the buttocks and are the strongest muscle group in the body. This stretch targets the area responsible for hip extension.

Lie down on the floor with one leg straight. Bend the knee of your other leg and bring it in toward your chest. Place your hands behind your knee and pull it in toward you to progressively increase the stretch. Make sure that your neck and shoulders are relaxed throughout the stretch and not raised off the floor. Hold the stretch for 15 seconds, then repeat on the other side.

Gluteus—Hip Rotated

This gluteus stretch targets the areas of the muscle group that extends and rotates the hip.

Lie down on the floor with both legs bent. Lift and externally rotate one leg, placing it over the other so that the outside of the ankle is resting on the knee of the other leg. Increase the stretch by placing hands around the thigh of the leg that is not rotated and pulling it in toward you. Hold the stretch for 15 seconds and then repeat on the other side.

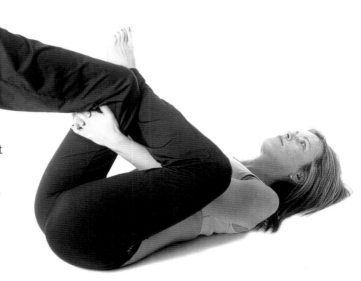

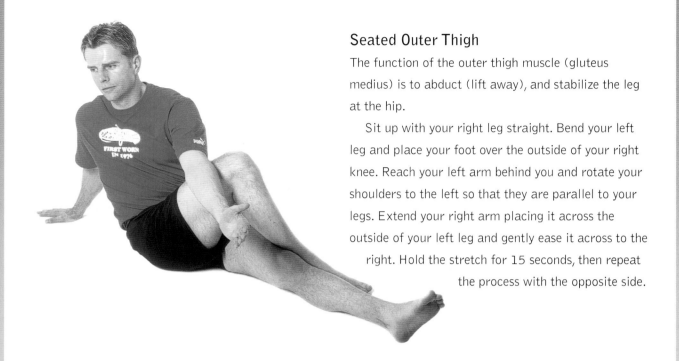

Seated Outer Thigh

The function of the outer thigh muscle (gluteus medius) is to abduct (lift away), and stabilize the leg at the hip.

Sit up with your right leg straight. Bend your left leg and place your foot over the outside of your right knee. Reach your left arm behind you and rotate your shoulders to the left so that they are parallel to your legs. Extend your right arm placing it across the outside of your left leg and gently ease it across to the right. Hold the stretch for 15 seconds, then repeat the process with the opposite side.

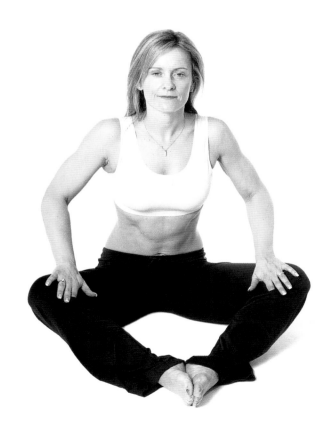

Seated Inner Thigh

The function of the inner thigh muscles (adductors) is to adduct (pull in), and stabilize the leg at the hip.

Sit up straight with both legs bent and externally rotated at the hip, with the soles of your feet touching. Using slight pressure from your arms, ease your knees down toward the floor. Hold the stretch for 15 seconds. Increase the pressure gradually each time you breathe out.

Standing Inner Thigh

This inner thigh (adductor) stretch targets a different area of the muscle group to the seated version, because the leg is extended.

Stand with your feet in a wide stance and turning out slightly. Keeping one leg straight, bend the knee of the other leg until you feel the stretch in the inner thigh of the straight one. Ensure that your hips and upper body remain straight. Hold the stretch for 15 seconds and then repeat on the other side.

Quadriceps

The quadriceps form a group of four muscles in the front of the thigh. They have various roles in the extension of the knee and flexion of the hip.

Position yourself standing on your right leg. Bend the knee of your left leg and take hold of your ankle with your left arm, lifting it up behind you so that your heel is near to your buttocks. Make sure that your body is completely straight with hips forward, legs close together, and knees in line. Aim to align your shoulder, hip, and knee to form a vertical line. Hold the stretch for 15 seconds and then repeat with your right leg.

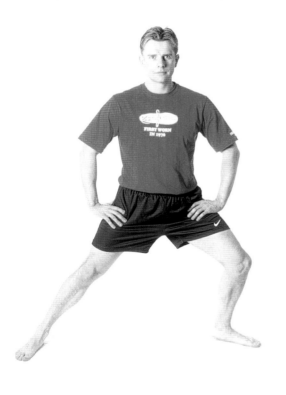

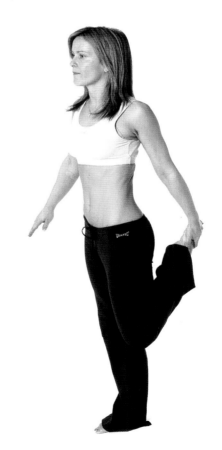

Hip Flexors

The group of muscles that flex the hip (hip flexors) have a valuable role in the control and stability of the hip. It is important for you to maintain a good level of flexibility in this muscle group to help prevent the onset of back pain caused by muscular imbalance.

Kneel down on your left knee with your body upright. Put your right foot forward and then progressively bend your right knee until you feel a stretch in the front and your hip and thigh of your left leg. Keep your shoulders and hips facing forward throughout the stretch. Hold for 15 seconds and then repeat with your right leg.

Gastrocnemius

The Gastrocnemius, normally referred to as the calf, is located at the back of the lower leg. Its main role is to planter flex the foot (to push the ball of the foot down) when your leg is straight.

Start by standing about a foot away from a wall or another sturdy object. Lean in and place your hands against the wall for support. Take a large step back with one leg keeping it straight. Slowly bend the knee of the leading leg until you feel a stretch in the back and bottom of the straight leg. Keep shoulders and hips parallel to the wall, feet pointing forward and back heel down throughout the stretch. Hold for 15 seconds and then repeat with your other leg.

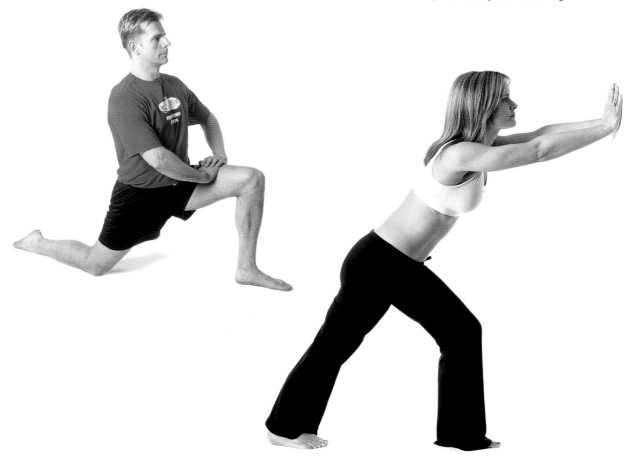

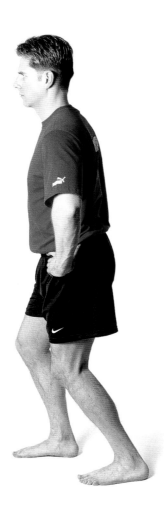

Soleus

The Soleus, also often referred to as the calf, is located below the Gastrocnemius at the back of the lower leg. Its main role is to planter flex the foot (to push the ball of the foot down) when the leg is bent at the knee.

Position yourself as in the Gastrocnemius stretch but away from the wall. Bring feet slightly closer together with both heels on the floor, and then slowly bend both knees until you feel tightening in the lower part of the back leg. Keep your body upright with shoulders and hips facing forward. Hold the stretch for 15 seconds and then repeat with the other leg.

Lower Back

The main function of muscles in the lower back is to support the spine via attachments to the pelvis; it is therefore highly beneficial to keep this area supple.

Lie on your back; bend your knees, bringing them up toward your chest. Place your arms behind your knees and gently pull them in close to your body. You can increase the area of the stretch by rolling your shoulders forward and tucking your head in. Hold the stretch for at least 15 seconds.

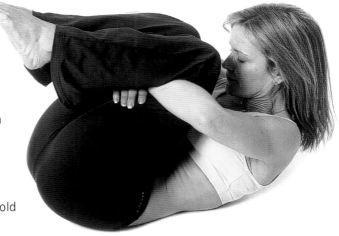

Sides

This stretch focuses on the external oblique and latissimus dorsi muscle groups in the side of the midsection and back.

Position yourself standing straight, with knees slightly bent. Reach one arm up, lifting your arm as high as possible, then laterally flex at the waist reaching your arm over and across in the same direction until you feel the stretch in your side. Hold this position for 15 seconds and then repeat on the other side. Make sure that you don't lean forward or backward during the stretch.

Upper Back

The upper back stretch targets the main muscle groups in the upper back and between your shoulders, with the main focus on the muscles between you shoulder blades—rhomboids. It also creates a secondary stretch in the forearms.

Stand with feet hip-width apart and knees slightly bent. Interlock fingers and rotate your wrists so that your palms are facing forward. Extend your arms pushing your hands forward until your arms are straight, round your shoulder to protract the shoulder blades and tilt your pelvis back very slightly. Hold the stretch for 15 seconds.

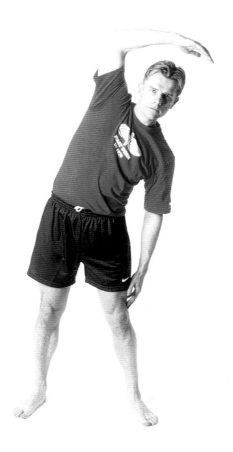
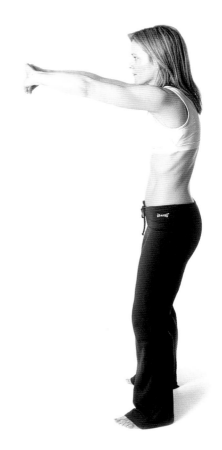

Chest

This stretch is a general chest stretch for the whole of the pectoral muscle group, and also lengthens the front of the shoulders (anterior deltoid).

Stand up straight with feet shoulder-width apart. Bend elbows to 90 degrees and raise your arms out to the side with hands in the air, until elbows are at shoulder height. Pull elbows behind, retracting your shoulders and sticking out your chest until you feel a stretch across your chest and in the front of your shoulders. Hold the stretch for 15 seconds.

Posterior Deltoid

This stretch focuses on the posterior deltoid, which is located at the back of the shoulders.

Stand straight, ideally with feet hip-width apart and shoulders facing forward. Bring one arm across your chest toward the opposite shoulder. Place your other hand just above the elbow and ease your upper arm toward your chest. Make sure that you don't rotate your upper body during the stretch. Hold this position for 15 seconds and then repeat on the other side.

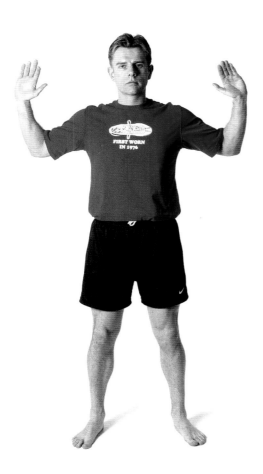

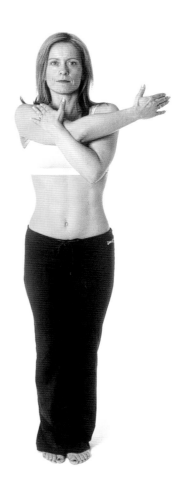

Triceps

The triceps are located in the back of the upper arm and can be quite difficult to stretch. This exercise provides the best overall stretch for the triceps group.

Stand straight with legs slightly bent at the knee. Raise one arm up above your head, bend it at the elbow, and place your hand behind you, touching between your shoulder blades. Lift the other arm above your head and cup your hand just above the elbow of the first arm. Ease the first arm back until you feel the stretch in the back of the upper arm. Hold this stretch for 15 seconds and then repeat with your other arm.

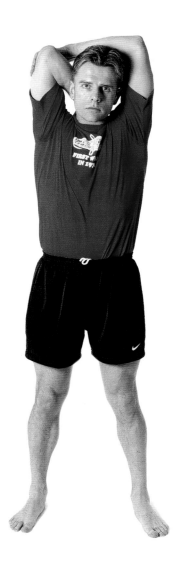

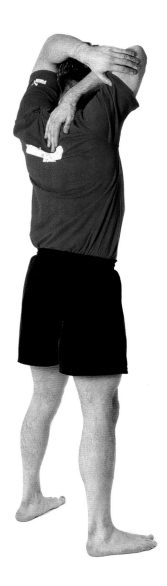

Biceps

The biceps muscle group is located in the front of the upper arm. This stretch targets the general biceps area, as well as the upper forearm.

Position yourself, ideally with feet shoulder width apart and body straight. Elevate both arms out to the side of your body and pull them back. Rotate your wrists inward until your palms are facing up and you feel a stretch in your biceps and upper forearm. Hold the stretch for 15 seconds.

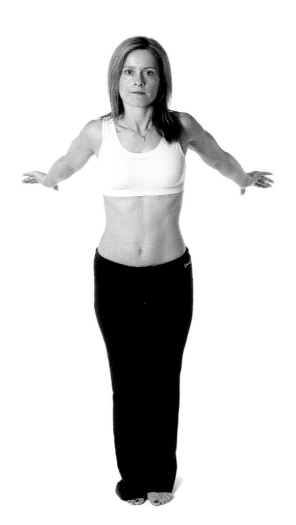

Combined Upper Body Stretch

This final stretch is a great combination stretch for the upper body. Its main focus areas are the chest (pectorals), front of shoulders (anterior deltoid), and sides of back (latissimus dorsi).

Kneel down on the floor, lean your torso forward with your arms extended above your head and hands flat on the floor. Lower your head between your shoulders and then slowly sit down onto your heel, pulling back against your hands.

Keeping shoulders low and hips straight, slowly walk both hands around, reaching to one side so that you are laterally flexing at the waist. Hold this position for 15 seconds, then walk your hands back to the center and repeat on the other side holding the stretch again for 15 seconds.

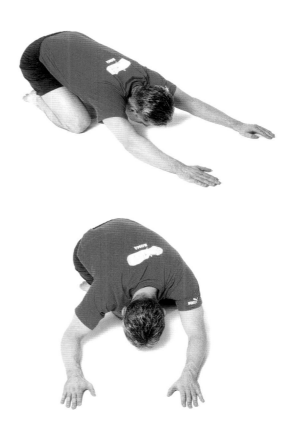

Exercises

Chest Press
Chest

This is a multiple joint exercise designed to work the major muscle groups in the front of the upper body in a forward pushing movement.

Attach the resistance band to a door anchor, or around a sturdy object of a suitable height (e.g. a pole), ensuring that it is positioned at shoulder height.

Position yourself with the band coming from behind you, your feet in a split stance, and leaning forward slightly with abdominal muscles tight. Hold the handles of the band in each hand with an overhand grip and elbows bent at 90 degrees. Ensure that elbows and wrists are all elevated to shoulder height and are parallel to the floor.

Extend both arms forward until they are straight and then slowly bend arms back to the start position, stopping when you feel a slight stretch across your chest and shoulders. To make the exercise harder step further forward, or make it easier by moving closer to the attachment.

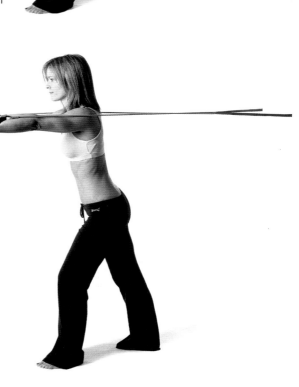

Muscle groups worked in this exercise: Chest (pectorals), front of shoulders (anterior deltoid), and back of upper arms (triceps).

Breathing tip: Breathe out as you extend arms forward.

Incline Chest Press

Chest

This is a multiple joint exercise designed to work the major muscle groups in the upper body in a forward and upward pushing movement.

Attach the resistance band to a door anchor, or around a sturdy object ensuring that it is positioned at waist height.

Position yourself, as in the standard Chest Press exercise, with the band coming from behind you, your feet in a split stance, and lean forward slightly with abdominal muscles tight. Hold the handles of the band in each hand, with elbows crooked at 90 degrees. Ensure that both forearms and wrists are elevated at a 40-degree angle to your shoulders and parallel to the angle of the band.

Extend both arms forward and up to just above head level, maintaining the 40-degree angle and until arms are straight, then slowly bend arms back to the start position, stopping when you feel a slight stretch across your chest and shoulders.

Muscle groups worked in this exercise: Upper chest (upper pectorals), front/middle of shoulders (anterior deltoid and medial deltoids), and back of upper arms (triceps).

Breathing tip: Breathe out as you extend arms forward.

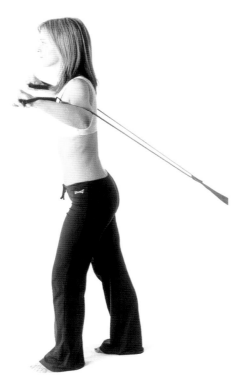
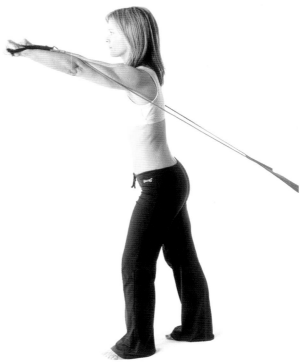

Decline Chest Press
Chest

This is a multiple joint exercise designed to work the major muscle groups in the front of the upper body in a forward and downward pushing movement.

Attach the resistance band to a door anchor, or around a sturdy object, ensuring that it is positioned just above head height.

Position yourself, as in the standard Chest Press exercise, with the band coming from behind you, your feet in a split stance, and leaning forward slightly with abdominal muscles tight. Hold the handles of the band in each hand with elbows bent at 90 degrees and elbows at shoulder height. Ensure that both forearms and wrists are lowered at a 40-degree angle to your shoulders and parallel to the angle of the band.

Extend both arms forward and down to waist level maintaining the 40-degree angle and until arms are straight, then slowly bend arms back to the start position, stopping when you feel a slight stretch across your chest and shoulders.

Muscle groups worked in this exercise: Lower chest (lower pectorals), front of shoulders (anterior deltoid), and back of upper arms (triceps).
Breathing tip: Breathe out as you extend arms forward.

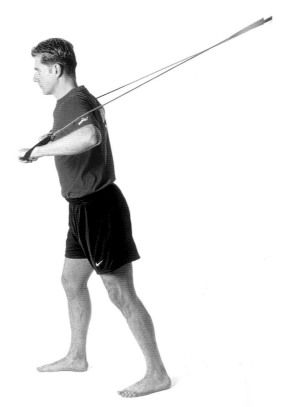
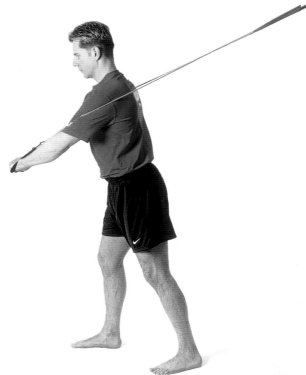

Single Arm Chest Flys

Chest

This is a single joint exercise designed to isolate the primary muscles of the chest and front of shoulder, in a shoulder and arm adduction movement.

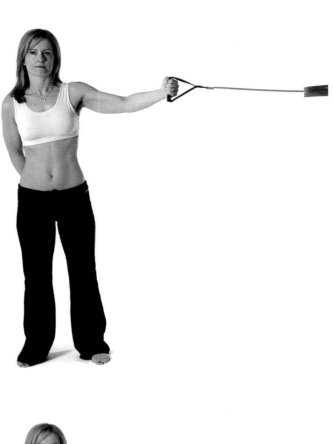

Attach the resistance band to a door anchor, or around a sturdy object, ensuring that it is positioned at shoulder height. You only need the use of one end of the band for this exercise, so ensure that the other end is securely attached to the anchor point.

Position yourself in the correct standing exercise posture, with your feet hip-width apart. The band should be on the side that you are working. From this position take hold of the handle with your arm extended out to the side and at shoulder height. Ensure that your elbow is pointing behind you and rotate your wrist so that the palm of your hand is facing forward. Slowly rotate your body away from the band until you feel resistance against your chest and shoulder.

Working against the resistance, bring your arm across in front of you, to just past mid-chest level, maintaining a slight bend in the elbow throughout the full range of the movement. Then slowly back to the starting position, stopping when you feel a slight stretch across your chest and shoulder. Your shoulders should remain parallel to your hips throughout the exercise to ensure that you don't rotate your upper body.

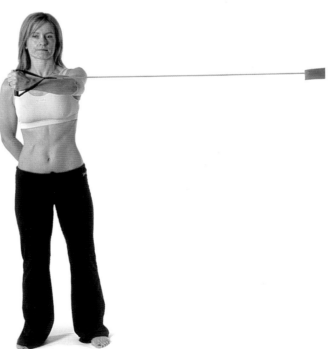

Muscle groups worked in this exercise: Chest (pectorals), front of shoulder (anterior deltoid).
Breathing tip: Breathe out as you bring your arm across in front of you.

Latissimus Pull Down
Upper Back

This is a multiple joint exercise designed to work the major muscle groups in the back of your upper body in a wide body pull-up movement.

Attach the resistance band to a door anchor, or around a sturdy object of a suitable height (e.g. a pole or beam) ensuring that it is positioned above head height.

Position yourself kneeling down facing the anchor point with the band coming from above you. Keeping your back straight and abdominal muscles tight to help support this posture, hold the handles of the band in each hand with palms facing forward and arms extended toward the anchor point.

Pull the band down in a straight line by bending arms, keeping a wide arm position, until your elbows pass the line of your back and reach your sides. You should feel a slight stretch across your chest — if not ensure that you are squeezing shoulder blades together at the bottom of the movement. Then extend your arms following the same line, until they are back to the start position. At this point they should be fully extended before beginning your next repetition. Check that your back remains straight and still throughout the exercise and prevent any swaying back and forth.

Muscle groups worked in this exercise: Back (latissimus dorsi), back of shoulders (posterior deltoid), and front of upper arms (biceps).
Breathing tip: Breathe out as you pull down.

Close Grip Pull Down

Upper Back

This is a multiple joint exercise designed to work the major muscle groups in the back of the upper body in a close arm pull-up movement, with slightly more emphasis on the arms than the Latissimus Pull Down.

Attach the resistance band to a door anchor, or around a sturdy object of a suitable height ensuring that it is positioned above head height.

Position yourself kneeling down facing the anchor point with the band coming from above you. Keeping your back straight and abdominal muscles tight to help support this posture, hold the handles of the band in each hand with palms facing each other and arms extended toward the anchor point. Ensure that your hands are approximately 6-8 inches (15-20cms) apart.

Pull the band down in a straight line by bending both arms, maintaining the close hand position with elbows in tight, until they reach your sides and hands touch your chest. You may feel a slight stretch across your chest. Then extend your arms following the same line, until they are back to the start position. At this point they should be fully extended before beginning your next repetition. Ensure that your back remains straight and still throughout the exercise to prevent any swaying back and forth.

Muscle groups worked in this exercise: Back (latissimus dorsi), back of shoulders (posterior deltoid), and front of upper arms (biceps).
Breathing tip: Breathe out as you pull down.

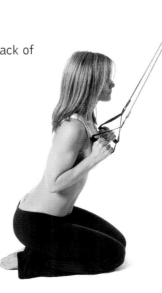

Standing Mid Row

Upper Back

This is a multiple joint exercise designed to work the major muscle groups in the upper back in a pulling/rowing movement.

   Attach the resistance band to a door anchor, or around a sturdy object of a suitable height ensuring that it is positioned at around shoulder height. Position yourself with the band in front of you, your feet in a split stance and body upright, with abdominal muscles tight. Hold the handles of the band with palms facing down and arms extended forward until they are straight. Elbows and wrists should be elevated to shoulder height and parallel to the floor.

   Slowly bend elbows pulling them back past the line of your shoulders, ensuring that elbows and wrists remain elevated to shoulder height and parallel to the floor. Then slowly straighten your arms back to the start position, stopping when they are fully extended. To make the exercise harder step further back, or make it easier by moving closer to the attachment.

Muscle groups worked in this exercise: Upper back (lower trapezius), back of shoulders (posterior deltoid), between shoulders (rhomboids), and front of upper arms (biceps).

Breathing tip: Breathe out as you pull arms backward.

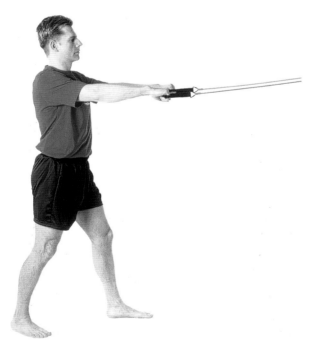 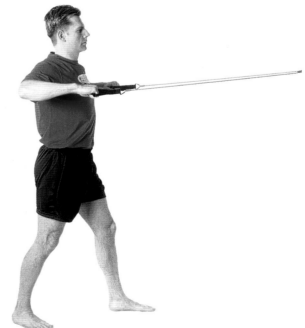

Bent Over Row

Upper Back

This is a multiple joint exercise and an alternative to the Mid Row, designed to work the major muscle groups in the upper back in a pulling/rowing movement.

Place the resistance band under the arches of both feet. Position yourself with feet shoulder-width apart, a slight bend in the knees and bent forward at the waist. The lumbar region of your back should be straight and not arched over. Keep abdominal muscles tight. Hold the handles of the band and extend your arms down toward the floor until they are straight and vertical.

With an overhand grip, bend elbows, pulling them back past the line of your shoulders, retracting shoulder blades and keeping your forearms vertical. Then slowly straighten your arms back to the start position, stopping when they are fully extended. Ensure that your back remains still throughout the exercise and prevent any swaying back and forth. You can move feet wider apart to make the exercise harder, or closer to make it easier.

Muscle groups worked in this exercise: Upper back (lower trapezius), back of shoulders (posterior deltoid), between shoulders (rhomboids), and front of upper arms (biceps).

Breathing tip: Breathe out as you pull arms up.

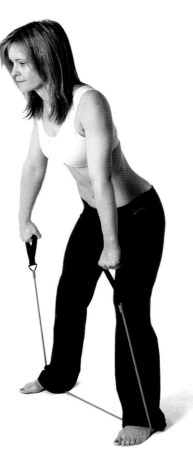
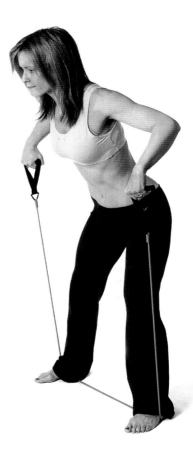

Band Pull Over
Back

This is a single joint isolation exercise designed to work the muscle groups in the middle/side of the back and assisted by those in the lower chest. These muscles are used in a movement similar to closing a large pull-down window.

Attach the resistance band to a door anchor, or around a sturdy object of a suitable height, ensuring that it is positioned just above floor level.

Position yourself lying flat on your back so that the anchor point is above your head. You can bend your knees to take the pressure off your lower back. Take hold of both handles with an underhand grip and extend them above your head, keeping them shoulder-width apart and near to the floor. When arms are extended, check that your lower back is flat on the floor and abdominal muscles are tight. This will help prevent any unwanted arching.

With tension already in the band, pull the band over and down, creating a large arc until your hands reach the side of your legs. Pause, and then slowly allow your arms to return back up and over following the same line, until they are back to the start position.

Muscle groups worked in this exercise: Back (latissimus dorsi) and lower chest (lower pectorals).
Breathing tip: Breathe out as you pull down.

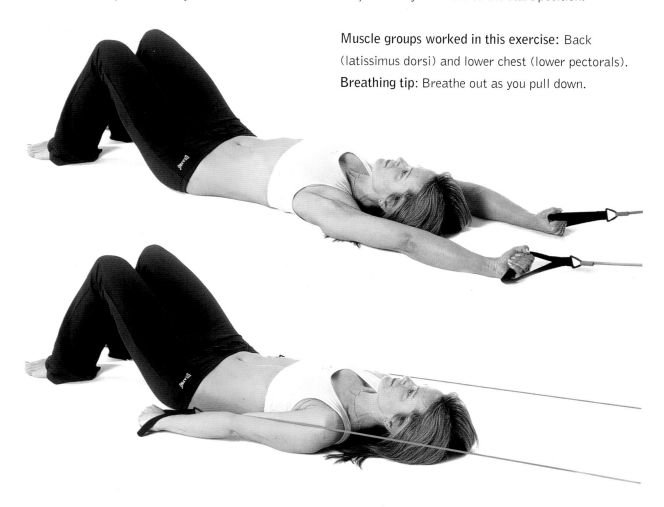

Upright Row
Shoulders

This is a multiple joint exercise designed to work the major muscle groups in the upper back and shoulders in an upright, arm lifting movement.

Place the resistance band under the arches of both feet. Position yourself with feet hip-width apart, and in the correct standing exercise posture. Keep abdominal muscles tight. Swap the handles of the band to opposite hands so that it crosses over and hold the handles with a close overhand grip. Extend arms down toward the floor until they are straight, but don't round your shoulders.

With elbows leading, lift the handles of the band until your hands reach your chin, keeping them as close to your body as possible throughout the movement. Elbows should be high and form a "V" with shoulder blades retracted. Then, slowly straighten your arms back to the start position, stopping when they are fully extended. Ensure that your back remains still throughout the exercise to prevent any swaying back and forth. You can keep feet wider apart to make the exercise harder, or closer to make it easier.

Muscle groups worked in this exercise: Upper back/neck (upper and lower trapezius), front and middle of shoulder (anterior and medial deltoid), and front of upper arms (biceps).

Breathing tip: Breathe out as you pull arms up.

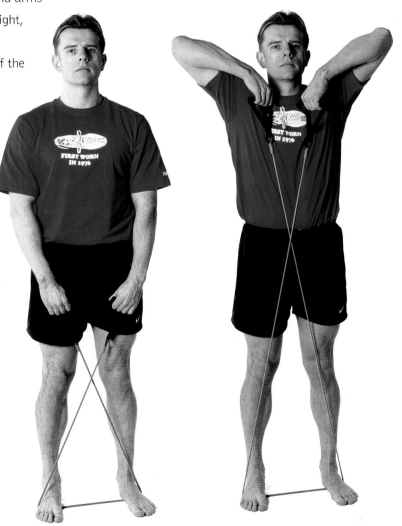

Shoulder Press
Shoulders

This is a multiple joint exercise designed to work the major muscle groups in the top of the shoulder and the back of the upper arm, in an upward pushing movement.

Place the resistance band on top of a swiss ball or chair and position yourself so that you are seated on top of the band. Sit straight with shoulders back and abdominal muscles tight. Using an overhand grip, hold the handles of the band with your hands to the side of each shoulder at around shoulder height.

Extend both arms above your head until they are straight and then slowly bend your arms taking them back to the start position, with your hands returning level with your shoulders. Make sure that your forearms remain vertical throughout the movement.

Muscle groups worked in this exercise: Front of shoulders (anterior deltoid), top of shoulders (upper trapezius) and back of upper arms (triceps).
Breathing tip: Breathe out as you extend arms up.

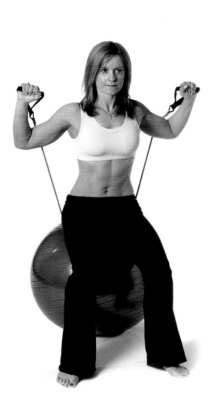
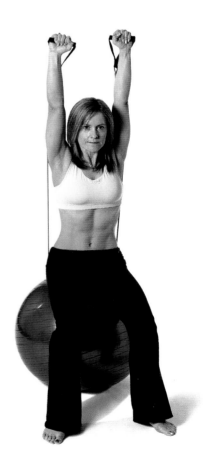

Lateral Raise

Shoulders

This is a single joint exercise designed to isolate the muscles in the middle of the shoulder in a lateral arm elevation movement.

Place the resistance band under the arches of both feet. Position yourself with feet hip-width apart and in the correct standing exercise posture. Keep abdominal muscles tight. Take hold of the handles with an overhand grip, palms facing inward and arms straight by your side.

Slowly elevate your arms up and out to the side, until your hands are just above shoulder height, pause, and then slowly bring arms back to the starting position, keeping arms extended. Ensure that your back remains still throughout the exercise to prevent any swaying or throwing of weight. To make the exercise harder, move feet further apart, or make it easier by moving them closer together.

Muscle group worked in this exercise: Middle of shoulder (medial deltoid).
Breathing tip: Breathe out as you bring your arms out to the side.

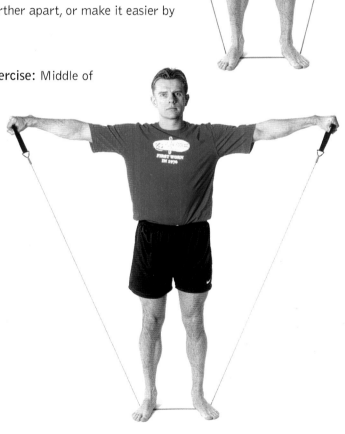

Single Arm Lateral Raise

Shoulders

This is an alternative single joint exercise that allows you to focus on one side at a time. It's designed to isolate the muscle in the middle of the shoulder in a lateral arm elevation movement.

Attach the resistance band to a door anchor, or around a sturdy object, ensuring that it is positioned at floor level. You only need the use of one end of the band for this exercise, so ensure that the other end is securely attached to the anchor point.

Position yourself with feet in a split stance and in the correct standing exercise posture. Keep abdominal muscles tight. The band should be coming from the opposite side to which you are working. From this position bring the band across the front of your body, taking hold of the handle with an overhand grip, palm facing inward, and holding your arm straight by your side. There should be some resistance at this point.

Slowly elevate your arm up and out to the side, until your hand is just above shoulder height, pause, and then slowly bring your arm back to the starting position, keeping it extended. Repeat with the other arm. Ensure that your back remains still throughout the exercise and prevent any swaying or throwing of weight. To make the exercise harder, step further away from the anchor point, or make it easier by moving closer.

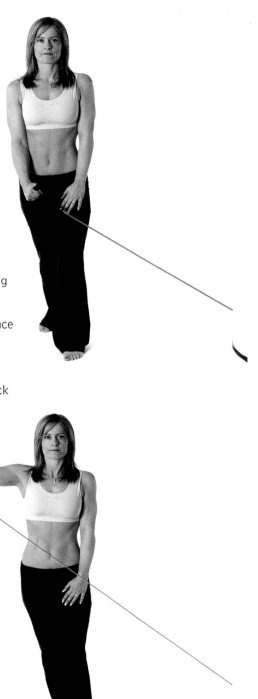

Muscle group worked in this exercise: Middle of shoulder (medial deltoid).

Breathing tip: Breathe out as you bring your arm out to the side.

Shoulder Front Raise
Shoulders

This is a single joint exercise designed to isolate the muscles in the front of the shoulder in a forward arm elevation movement.

Place the resistance band under the arches of both feet. Position yourself with feet hip-width apart and in the correct standing exercise posture. Keep abdominal muscles tight. Take hold of the handles with an overhand grip and arms straight by your side.

Slowly elevate your arms up in front of you, until your hands are just above shoulder height, pause, and then slowly bring arms back to the starting position, keeping arms extended throughout the full range of movement. Ensure that your back remains still throughout the exercise and prevent any swaying or throwing of weight. To make the exercise harder, move feet further apart, or make it easier by moving them closer together.

Muscle group worked in this exercise: Front of shoulder (anterior deltoid).

Breathing tip: Breathe out as you bring your arms up.

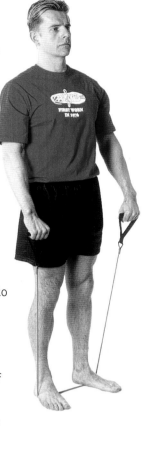

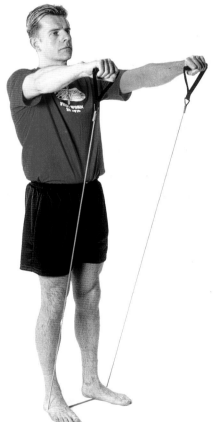

Single Arm Front Raise

Shoulders

This is an alternative single joint exercise that allows you to focus on one side at a time. It's designed to isolate the muscle in the front of the shoulder in a forward arm elevation movement.

Attach the resistance band to a door anchor, or around a sturdy object, such as a pole, ensuring that it is positioned at floor level. You only need the use of one end of the band for this exercise, so ensure that the other end is securely attached to the anchor point.

Position yourself so that the band is coming from behind you, with feet in a split stance, and in the correct standing exercise posture. Keep abdominal muscles tight. Take hold of the handle with an overhand grip and arm straight by your side.

Slowly elevate your arm up in front of you, until your hand is just above shoulder height, pause, and then slowly bring it back to the starting position, keeping your arm extended throughout the full range of movement. Then repeat using the other arm. Ensure that your back remains still throughout the exercise and prevent any swaying or throwing of weight. To make the exercise harder, step further away from the anchor point, or make it easier by moving closer.

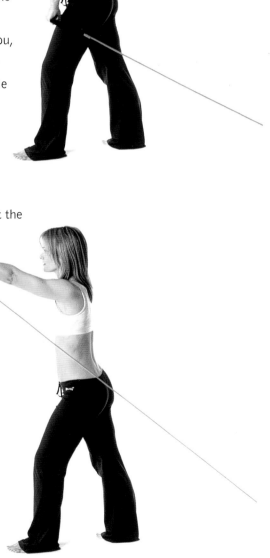

Muscle group worked in this exercise: Front of shoulder (anterior deltoid).

Breathing tip: Breathe out as you bring your arm up.

Reverse Flys

Shoulders

This is a single joint exercise designed to isolate the muscles at the back of the shoulder in a shoulder blade adduction/pulling-arms-to-the-rear movement. This is an area commonly neglected in training and everyday activities; it is therefore an important area to include in your program.

Attach the resistance band to a door anchor, or around a sturdy object, ensuring that it is positioned at shoulder height.

Position yourself with the band in front of you and in the correct standing exercise posture, with your feet in a split stance. Take hold of the handles with a palms-inward grip, your arms extended forward at shoulder height, and a very slight bend in the elbows. There should be tension in the band already.

Working against the resistance, bring your arms apart and out to the side keeping arms at shoulder height. Retract shoulder blades together, pause, and then slowly bring arms back to the starting position, with arms extended. Ensure that your back remains still throughout the exercise and prevent any swaying or throwing of weight. To make the exercise harder, step further back or make it easier by moving closer to the attachment.

Muscle groups worked in this exercise: Back of shoulder (posterior deltoid) and between shoulder blades (rhomboids).

Breathing tip: Breathe out as you bring your arms out to the side.

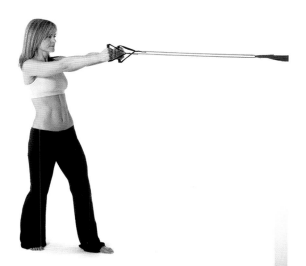

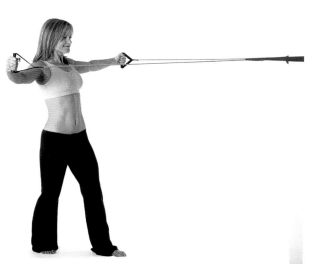

Rotator Cuff

The Rotator Cuff is a group of four muscles located at the front, top, and back of the shoulder joint originating from the shoulder blade. They are responsible for creating outward, inward, and upward circular motion or rotation in the shoulder. The following exercises will help you to create strength in the shoulder joint and prevent shoulder instability. These exercises are especially beneficial to those who play sports that require overarm motions, such as serving in tennis.

Lying Internal Shoulder Rotation

Rotator Cuff

This is a single joint isolation exercise designed to work the muscle group that stabilizes the shoulder joint. The muscles worked in this exercise are typically recruited in racket sports and when performing an overarm throwing action.

Attach the resistance band to a door anchor, or around a sturdy object of a suitable height, ensuring that it is positioned at floor level. You will only be using one handle.

Position yourself lying flat on your back so that the anchor point is above your head. You can bend your knees to take the pressure off your lower back. Take hold of the handle with an underhand grip, bending arm at the elbow. Position your upper arm so that it is at 90 degrees to your body with your shoulder and elbow touching the floor. Slowly rotate your shoulder allowing your hand to move down toward the floor at head height and as far as you can comfortably go. There should not be any pain. If pain is present, raise your hand away from the floor slightly. This is the correct starting position.

With tension already in the band, rotate your shoulder by lifting your hand up and over in an arc, pivoting on the elbow. Rotate as far as is comfortable and without the shoulder lifting away from the floor. Pause, and then slowly allow your shoulder to rotate back by lifting your hand back up and over, following the same line, until it is back to the start position. Make sure your upper arm and elbow stay fixed in position. Repeat using your other hand.

Muscle group worked in this exercise: Rotator cuff.
Breathing tip: Breathe out as you move your hand in the direction of your feet.

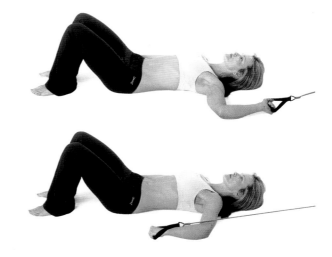

Lying External Shoulder Rotation
Rotator Cuff

This is another highly beneficial single joint isolation exercise designed to work the muscle group that stabilizes the shoulder joint. The muscles worked in this exercise are typically recruited in racket sports when performing a backhand return shot, setting up for a serve, volley, and overarm throw.

Attach the resistance band to a door anchor, or around a sturdy object of a suitable height ensuring that it is positioned at floor level. You will only be using one handle.

Position yourself lying flat on your back so that the anchor point is by your feet. As before, you can bend your knees to take the pressure off your lower back. Take hold of the handle with an overhand grip, bending your arm at the elbow. Position your upper arm so that it is at 90 degrees to your body with your shoulder and elbow touching the floor. Get into the start position by rotating your shoulder, allowing your

hand to move down toward the floor at waist height, and as far as it can comfortably go. There should not be any pain. If pain is present, raise your hand away from the floor slightly.

With tension already in the band, rotate your shoulder by lifting your hand up and over in an arc, pivoting on the elbow and stopping when it reaches the floor at head height. Pause, and then slowly allow your shoulder to rotate back by lifting your hand back up and over following the same line, until it is back to the start position. Make sure that your upper arm and elbow stay fixed in position and that your shoulder does not lift away from the floor throughout the exercise.

Muscle group worked in this exercise: Rotator cuff.
Breathing tip: Breathe out as you move your hand in the direction of your head.

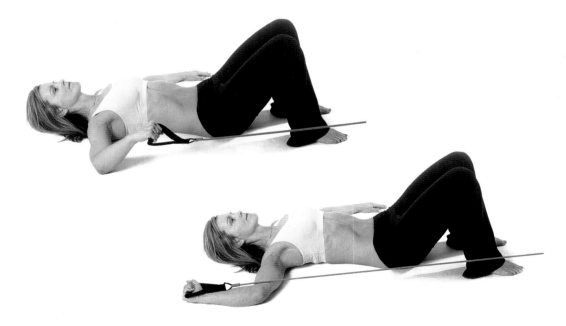

Standing External Shoulder Rotation
Rotator Cuff

This is an alternative single joint isolation exercise designed to work the muscle group that stabilizes the shoulder joint. The muscles worked in this exercise are typically used in racket sports when performing a backhand return shot, setting up for a serve, or playing golf.

Attach the resistance band to a door anchor, or around a sturdy object of a suitable height ensuring that it is positioned at elbow height. You will only be using one handle.

Position yourself in the correct exercise posture sideways on to the anchor point, with the band on the opposite side to the one that you're working. Take hold of the handle with a palm-in grip, bending the arm 90 degrees at the elbow. Position your upper arm so that it is tight to your body. Get into the start position by rotating your shoulder so that your forearm is across your body.

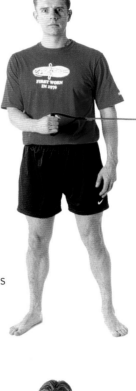

With tension already in the band, rotate your shoulder by swinging your arm around to the side, pivoting your elbow on your hip, and stopping when it is parallel with the band. Pause, and then slowly allow your shoulder to rotate back by swinging your arm back across your body, following the same line, and until it reaches the start position. Make sure that your upper arm and elbow stay fixed in position and that your shoulders and midsection don't sway during the exercise.

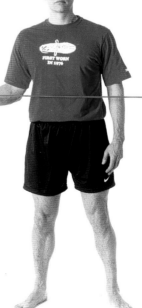

Muscle group worked in this exercise: Rotator cuff.
Breathing tip: Breathe out as you move your arm out to the side.

Bicep Curls

Arms

This is a single joint exercise designed to isolate the muscles in the front of the upper arms in a hand lifting movement flexing at the elbow.

Place the resistance band under the arches of both feet. Position yourself with feet hip-width apart, and in the correct standing exercise posture. Keep abdominal muscles tight. Take hold of the handles with an under-hand grip, and arms straight by your side.

Slowly elevate your hands in front of you by flexing at the elbow, keeping a strict position with the upper arms locked by your sides. Pause when your hands are at chest height, but not touching your chest, and then slowly straighten arms back down to the starting position, stopping when your hands reach the side of your legs. Ensure that your back and upper arms remain still throughout the exercise to prevent any swaying. To make the exercise harder, move feet further apart, or make it easier by moving them closer together.

Muscle group worked in this exercise: Front of upper arms (biceps).

Breathing tip: Breathe out as you bring your hands up.

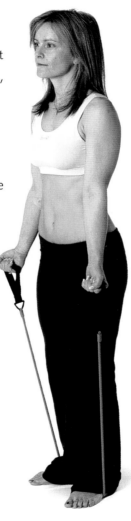
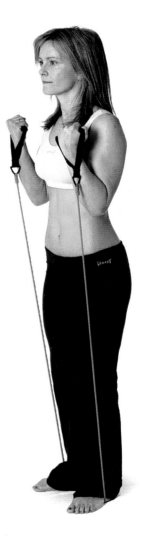

Individual Bicep Curls

Arms

This is an alternative to the standard bicep curl, allowing you to concentrate on working each arm individually, though it is more time consuming.

Place the resistance band under the arches of both feet. Position yourself with feet hip-width apart, and in the correct standing exercise posture. Keep abdominal muscles tight. Take hold of the handles with an under-hand grip, and arms straight by your side.

Slowly elevate one arm in front of you by flexing at the elbow, keeping a strict position with the upper arm locked by your sides. Pause when your hand is at shoulder height, but not touching your shoulder, and then slowly straighten arm back to the starting position, stopping when your hand reaches the side of your leg. Ensure that your back and upper arms remain still throughout the exercise to prevent any swaying or throwing of weight. Repeat with the other arm. To make the exercise harder, move feet further apart, or make it easier by moving them closer together.

Muscle group worked in this exercise: Front of upper arms (biceps).

Breathing tip: Breathe out as you bring your hands up.

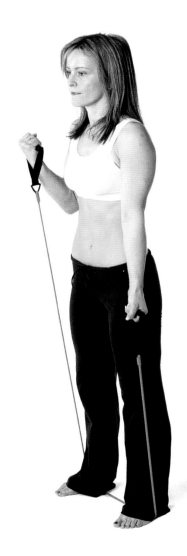

Bicep Hammer Curls

Arms

This is a similar single joint exercise to the standard Bicep Curl, putting additional emphasis on the forearm in a hand-lifting movement when flexing at the elbow.

Place the resistance band under the arches of both feet. Position yourself with feet hip-width apart, and in the correct standing exercise posture. Keep abdominal muscles tight. Take hold of the handles with a palms-in grip and arms straight by your side.

Slowly elevate your hands in front of you by flexing at the elbow, keeping palms facing in and a strict position with the upper arms locked by your sides. Pause when your hands are at shoulder height, but not touching your shoulders, and then slowly straighten arms back to the starting position, stopping when your hands reach the side of your legs. Ensure that your back and upper arms remain still throughout the exercise to prevent any swaying or throwing of weight. To make the exercise harder, push feet further apart, or make it easier by moving them closer together.

Muscle group worked in this exercise: Front of upper arms (biceps).

Breathing tip: Breathe out as you bring your hands up.

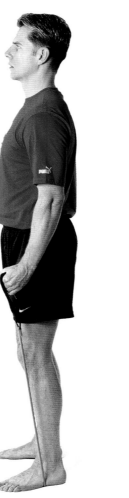 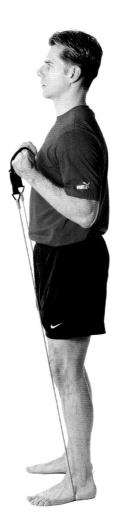

Tricep Extension

Arms

This is a single joint exercise designed to isolate the muscles in the back of the upper arms in a reaching-out movement, when extending at the elbow and pulling down.

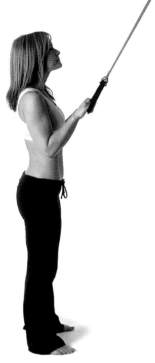

Attach the resistance band to a door anchor, or around a sturdy object of a suitable height (e.g. a pole), ensuring that it is as far as possible above head height.

Position yourself so that the band is as vertical as possible, with feet hip-width apart, and in the correct standing exercise posture. Keep abdominal muscles tight. Take hold of the handles with an overhand grip and with elbows locked in by your sides, bend your arms until hands are at shoulder height.

Slowly extend your arms pushing the handles down until they touch your thighs, pause, and then bend your arms returning your hands back to the start position. Ensure that you keep your upper arm and elbows fixed by your sides and do not let them spring out. Keep shoulders and back still throughout the exercise to prevent any swaying or throwing of weight.

Muscle group worked in this exercise: Back of upper arms (triceps).
Breathing tip: Breathe out as you straighten arms.

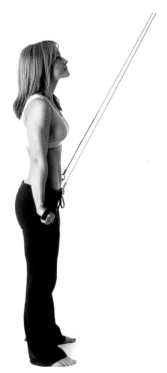

Tricep Overhead Extension
Arms

This triceps exercise is designed to isolate the muscles in the back of the upper arms and work it through a different angle to the previous triceps exercise. Muscle areas are used in a reaching-out movement, extending at the elbow, as if you were going to hit an object with a hammer.

Place the resistance band under one foot, standing on a part of the band that allows a good level of tension. Ensure that the band is coming out from the back of your foot. You only require one handle for this exercise.

Position yourself with feet in a close split stance and the band under your back foot. Keep abdominal muscles tight. With the band behind you, take hold of the handle with the opposite hand to the foot that is on the band, with an inverted palm-in grip. Extend your arm above your head, and then bend the elbow so that your forearm is behind your head. Keep upper arm vertical.

Slowly extend your arm pushing the handle up in the air until your arm is straight, pause, and then bend your arm returning your hands back to the start position. Ensure that you keep your upper arm vertical and still throughout the exercise. Repeat exercise with the other arm. Make sure that your neck is comfortable during the exercise by looking straight ahead and not craning it forward.

Muscle group worked in this exercise: Back of upper arms (triceps).

Breathing tip: Breathe out as you extend arm up.

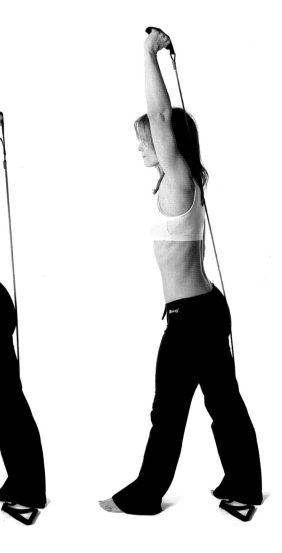

Triceps Kickbacks

Arms

This final triceps exercise is an alternative to the overhead Triceps extension, and can be more comfortable if you have a limited rage of movement in your shoulders. It also works the triceps under less tension.

Attach the resistance band to a door anchor, or around a sturdy object of a suitable height ensuring that it is positioned at floor level. Only one handle is required.

Position yourself with the resistance band in front of you, feet in a split stance, leaning your upper body forward to about 45 degrees. Rest the hand that you're not using on the thigh of your leading leg for support. Take hold of the handle with a palm-in grip; your upper arm should remain close to your side with elbow bent and then elevated to shoulder height.

Starting with your hand below your shoulder, slowly extend your arm, pulling the handle back behind you until your arm is straight, pause, and then bend your arm, returning your hand back to the start position. Ensure that you keep your upper arm horizontal and held in position throughout the exercise. Repeat exercise with the other arm. To make the exercise harder, step further away from the anchor point, or make it easier by moving closer.

Muscle group worked in this exercise: Back of upper arms (triceps).
Breathing tip: Breathe out as you extend arm back.

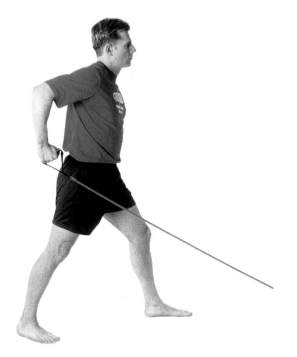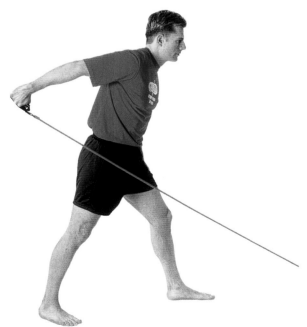

Squat

Legs & Hips

This is a multiple joint exercise designed to work the major muscle groups of the legs in the front of the thighs and buttocks. These groups are used in a seated to standing movement and when skiing.

Place the resistance band under the arches of both feet. Position yourself in the correct standing exercise posture, with feet shoulder-width apart. Take hold of the handles with an overhand grip and bring them up to shoulder level with the palm of your hands facing forward. The band should be behind your arms.

Slowly bend your knees keeping your heels down, and push your weight back slightly as if you were about to sit down, stopping just before your legs reach a 90-degree angle. Pause, and then extend your legs pushing through your heels until you are back to the starting position. Try to keep your back and lower legs as vertical as possible throughout the exercise. Avoid pushing your knees forward past the toe line as you bend your knees. You can move feet wider apart to make the exercise harder, or closer to make it easier.

Muscle groups worked in this exercise: Front of thigh (quadriceps), buttocks (gluteus maximus).
Breathing tip: Breathe out as you extend legs.

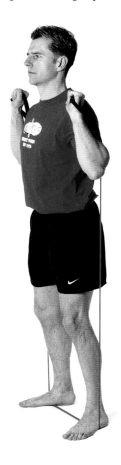

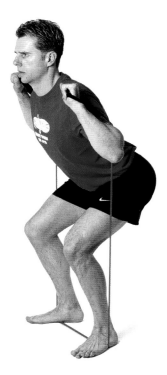

Lying Leg Extension

Legs & Hips

This is a single joint exercise designed to isolate the muscle group in the front of the upper leg in a forward leg kick action.

Using the ankle strap, attach the resistance band around the ankle of the leg that you're starting with.

Position yourself lying on your front, taking hold of both handles with your hands above your head and elbows firmly on the floor. Bend the knee of the leg you're exercising so that your foot is near to your buttocks.

Extend your leg at the knee, keeping the upper part of the leg still, until your leg is straight and your foot touches the floor. Pause, and then slowly bend the knee again, bringing your foot back to the starting position. Repeat using your other leg. Ensure that your hips remain still and keep knees together throughout the exercise.

Muscle group worked in this exercise: Front of thigh (quadriceps).

Breathing tip: Breathe out as you extend leg.

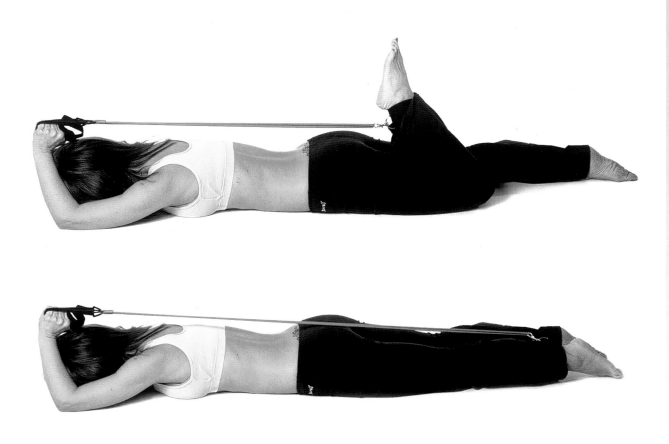

Standing Leg Extension

Legs & Hips

This is an alternative exercise to the Lying Leg Extension, designed to isolate the muscle group in the front of the upper leg.

Attach the resistance band to a door anchor, or around a sturdy object, ensuring that it is positioned at floor level. You only need to use one end of the band for this exercise, so ensure that the other end is secure. Attach the loose end to an ankle strap, and then place around the ankle of the leg that you are starting with.

Position yourself so that the band is coming from behind you and in the correct standing exercise posture. Stand on one leg, flexing the other at the hip so that the thigh is at 45 degrees. Bend the knee of the elevated leg so that your foot drops back. Keep abdominal muscles tight. Place a stable object next to you, to hold onto for support, if necessary.

Extend your leg at the knee, keeping the upper part of the leg still, until your leg is straight. Pause, and then slowly bend the knee again. Bring your foot back to the starting position. After completing your repetitions, swap legs. Ensure that your hips remain still throughout the exercise. To make the exercise harder, step further away from the anchor point, or make it easier by moving closer.

Muscle group worked in this exercise: Front of thigh (quadriceps).
Breathing tip: Breathe out as you extend leg.

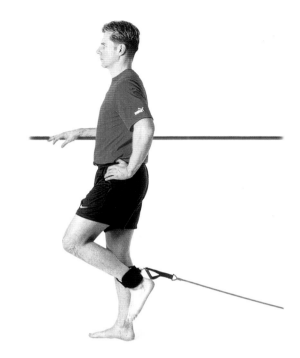

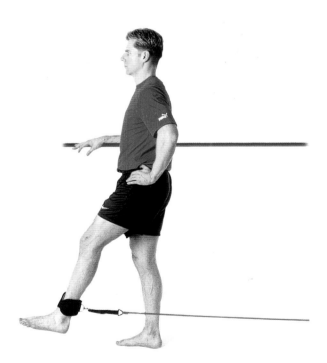

Lying Hamstring Curl

Legs & Hips

This is a single joint exercise designed to isolate the muscle group in the back of the upper leg.

Attach the resistance band to a door anchor, or around a sturdy object, ensuring that it is positioned at floor level. You only need to use one end of the band for this exercise, so ensure that the other end is secure. Attach the loose end to an ankle strap and then place around the ankle of the leg that you are starting with.

Position yourself lying on your front, with the band coming from behind your feet and both legs straight.

Bend the knee of the leg you're exercising until your heel is near to your buttocks. Pause, and then slowly extend your leg again. Bring it straight and back to the starting position. Repeat using your other leg. Ensure that your hips remain still and keep your knees together throughout the exercise.

Muscle group worked in this exercise: Back of upper leg (hamstrings).

Breathing tip: Breathe out as you bend the knee.

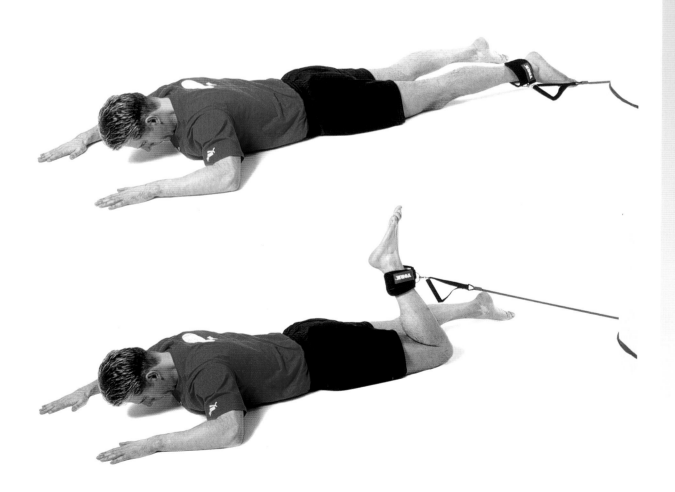

Standing Hamstring Curl
Legs & Hips

This is an alternative exercise to the Lying Hamstring Curl, designed to isolate the muscle group in the back of the upper leg.

Attach the resistance band to a door anchor, or around a sturdy object, ensuring that it is positioned at floor level. You only need to use one end of the band for this exercise, so ensure that the other end is secure. Attach the loose end to an ankle strap, and then place around the ankle of the leg that you are starting with.

Position yourself so that the band is coming from in front of you and in the correct standing exercise posture with knees in line. You can place a stable object next to you to hold onto for support.

Whilst supporting all your weight with one leg, flex the other at the knee until the lower leg is at 90 degrees to the upper. Pause, and then extend the leg at the knee until your leg is straight. Repeat using your other leg. Ensure that your hips remain still and keep both knees together throughout the exercise. To make the exercise harder, step further away from the anchor point, or make it easier by moving closer.

Muscle group worked in this exercise: Back of upper leg (hamstrings).
Breathing tip: Breathe out as you bend the knee.

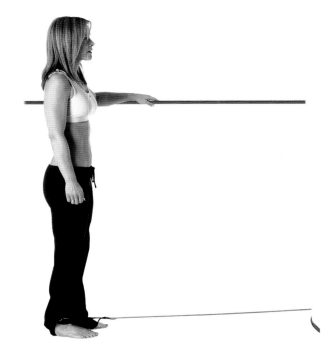

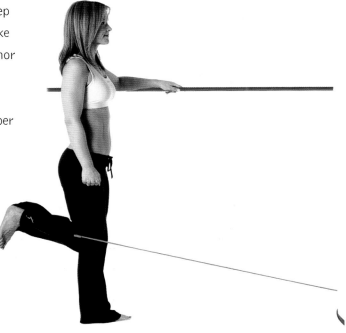

Calf Flex

Legs & Hips

This is an alternative calf exercise, designed for working one leg at a time. It isolates the major muscle group at the back of the lower leg.

Place both resistance band handles over the toes of one foot.

Position yourself in the correct standing exercise posture. Take hold of the middle of the band with an overhand grip and bring them up to chest level. Extend the leg with the band attached, so that it is straight and off the ground.

Keeping the leg straight, push your toes down against the band pivoting at the ankle, as if pushing on a brake pedal. Pause, and then lift your toes back as far as possible and to the start position. Repeat with the other leg. You can move hands wider apart to make the exercise harder or closer to make it easier.

Muscle groups worked in this exercise: Back of lower leg (calf).

Breathing tip: Breathe out as you push toes down.

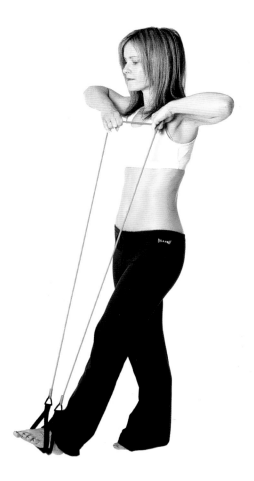
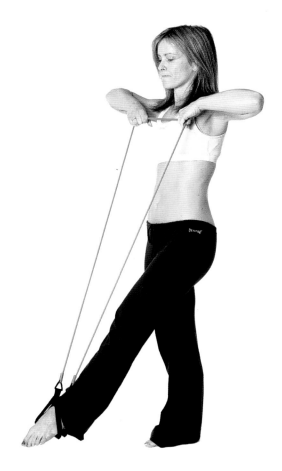

Lying Side Leg Raise

Legs & Hips

This is a single joint isolation exercise designed to work the muscle group that abducts the leg. This muscle has an important role in stabilizing the hip.

Tie the ends of the resistance band together so that it forms a loop, just over two feet (60cms) in diameter.

Position yourself lying on your side in a straight line with shoulders and hips vertical. Place both legs through the middle of the band so that it sits just above the knee. Slightly bend the leg that is on the floor for added support.

Keeping your foot flexed, lift (abduct) the top leg, aiming to get it to a 40- to 45-degree angle to the floor. Pause, and then slowly lower your leg back down until it reaches the start position, but not touching the other leg. Make sure that hips remain fixed during the exercise and that they don't rotate back when lifting your leg. Repeat using your other leg.

Muscle group worked in this exercise: Outer thigh/hip (gluteus medius).

Breathing tip: Breathe out as you lift leg up.

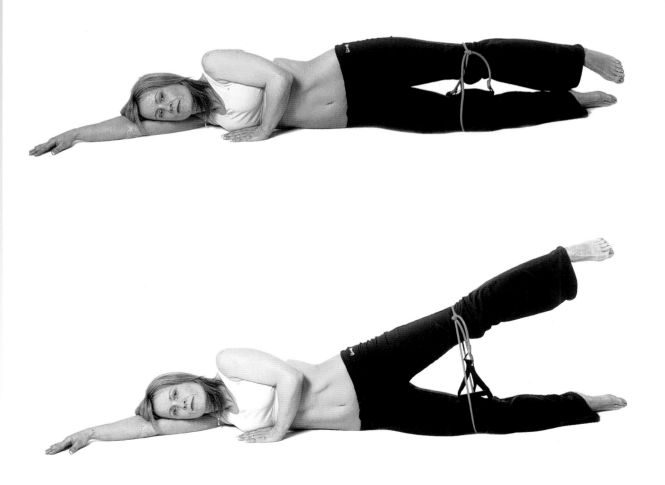

Standing Outer Thigh

Legs & Hips

This is an alternative single joint exercise to the Lying Side Leg Raise, providing the same benefits but in a standing position.

Attach the resistance band to a door anchor, or around a sturdy object, ensuring that it is positioned at floor level. You only need to use one end of the band for this exercise, so ensure that the other end is secure. Attach the loose end to an ankle strap, and then place around the ankle of the leg that you are starting with.

Position yourself in the correct standing exercise posture so that you are side on to the anchor point with the band attached to the leg that is furthest away. The leg that you are working should be slightly crossed over the front of the one that you are standing on. You can place a stable object next to you to hold onto for support.

Whilst supporting all your weight with one leg, lift (abduct) the other out to the side until it reaches a 40- to 45-degree angle. Pause, and then lower your leg until it crosses the supporting leg. Repeat using the other leg. Ensure that your leg is straight and the upper body remains still throughout the exercise to prevent any flexing of the waist. To make the exercise harder, step further away from the anchor point, or make it easier by moving closer.

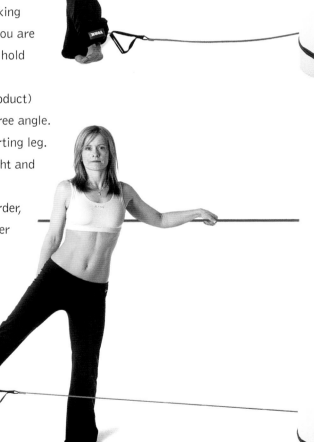

Muscle group worked in this exercise: Outer thigh/hip (gluteus medius).
Breathing tip: Breathe out as you lift leg out to the side.

Inner Thigh

Legs & Hips

This is a single joint isolation exercise designed to work the muscle group that adducts the leg. This muscle also has an important role in stabilizing the hip from the inner thigh.

Attach the resistance band to a door anchor, or around a sturdy object, ensuring that it is positioned at floor level. You only need to use one end of the band for this exercise, so ensure that the other end is secure.

Position yourself in the correct standing exercise posture so that you are side on to the anchor point. Attach the loose end of the band to an ankle strap, place it around the ankle of the leg that is closest to the anchor, and abduct (lift) your leg toward the anchor. You can place a stable object next to you to hold onto for support.

Whilst supporting all your weight with one leg, adduct the other, bringing it across the supporting leg. Pause, and then bring it back across and out to the side, returning to the start position. Repeat using the other leg. Ensure that your leg is straight, and your upper body remains still throughout the exercise to prevent any flexing at the waist. To make the exercise harder, step further away from the anchor point, or make it easier by moving closer.

Muscle group worked in this exercise: Inner thigh/hip (adductors).

Breathing tip: Breathe out as you bring leg in.

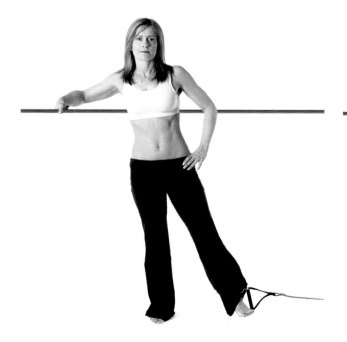
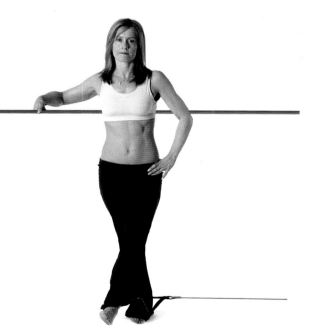

Lunge

Legs & Hips

This is a multiple joint exercise designed to work the major muscle groups of the legs in the front of the thighs and buttocks. These groups are worked in a seated to standing movement. It is similar to the squat, but enables you to focus on each leg individually.

Position yourself in the correct standing exercise posture, and then take a large step forward with one foot and place the band underneath it. Keep both legs extended, feet parallel, with your leading foot flat and the heel of your back foot raised. Hold the handles of the band with an overhand grip, and bring them up to shoulder level with the palm of your hands facing forward. The band should be behind your arms. Slowly bend your knees, stopping just before the knee of your back leg touches the floor, and both legs are bent to a 90-degree angle. Pause, and then extend your legs pushing through the heel of the leading leg until you are back to the start position. Try to keep your back as vertical as possible throughout the exercise. Ensure that the knee of your leading leg remains in line with your ankle as your knee bends.

Muscle groups worked in this exercise: Front of thigh (quadriceps), buttocks (gluteus maximus).
Breathing tip: Breathe out as you extend legs.

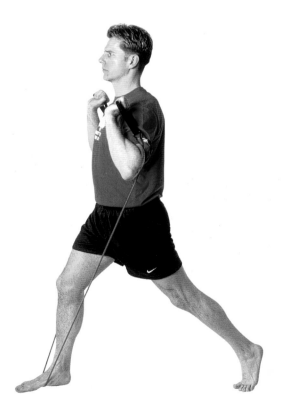
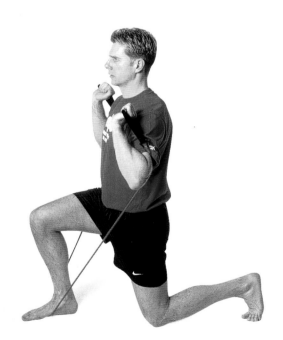

Hip/Leg Extension

Legs & Hips

This is a multiple joint exercise designed to work the major muscle group of the buttocks. This group is used in movements such as the pushing-down action when pedaling a bicycle. It activates similar areas to the squat, but with more emphasis on the buttocks.

Position yourself on your hands and knees, or elbows if it is more comfortable. Place the resistance band in the arch of one of your feet; take hold of both handles with a palms-in grip and with the band on the inside of your arms. Raise the knee of the side you are working toward your chest and make sure that your back is completely straight.

Slowly extend your hip and leg, pushing your foot directly behind you, stopping when it forms a straight line with your body and with your foot at hip height. Pause, and then flex your hip and bend your knee bringing it back toward your chest and to the start position. Abdominal muscles should be held tight to prevent your back from arching. Keep your foot fixed in position with toes down throughout the exercise to prevent the band from slipping off. Repeat on your other side.

Muscle group worked in this exercise: Buttocks (gluteus maximus).

Breathing tip: Breathe out as you extend hip leg.

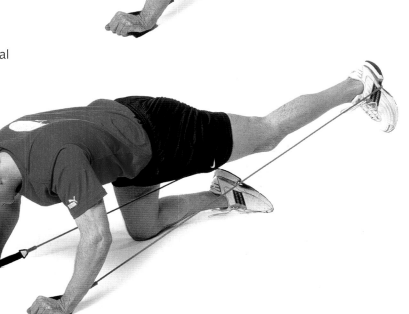

Hip Flexion

Legs & Hips

This is a single joint exercise, designed to isolate the muscle group in the front of the hip. This muscle group is typically used when lifting your knee toward your chest; it is therefore an important part of most sporting movements, especially running.

Attach the resistance band to a door anchor, or around a sturdy object, ensuring that it is positioned at floor level. You only need to use one end of the band for this exercise, so ensure that the other end is secure. Attach the loose end to an ankle strap and then place around the ankle of the leg that you are starting with.

Position yourself so that the band is coming from behind you and in the correct standing exercise posture. Stand on one leg, extending the other at the hip and knee so that the thigh is at 30 degrees behind you. Keep your body upright and abdominal muscles tight. Place a stable object next to you so that you can hold onto it for support.

In a forward movement flex your hip, allow the knee to bend, and lift the knee as high as possible toward your chest without moving your back out of the upright position. Pause, and then slowly lower your knee, extending your hip and leg back to the starting position. Repeat using the other leg. Ensure that your upper body remains still throughout the exercise. To make the exercise harder, step further away from the anchor point, or make it easier by moving closer.

Muscle group worked in this exercise: Hip flexors (iliopsoas).

Breathing tip: Breathe out as you lift knee.

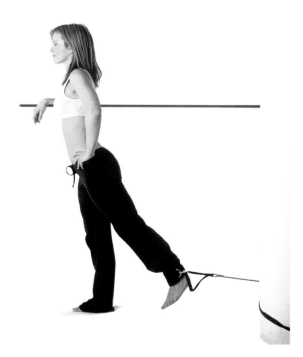
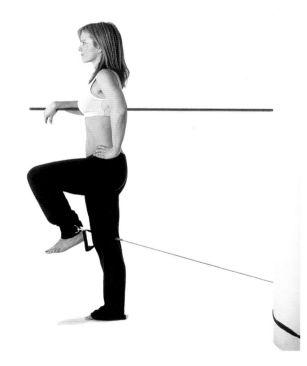

Abdominal Curl

Midsection

To provide a fully-balanced workout, some exercises are needed that don't require a resistance band. This is a basic, yet effective, exercise designed to work the major muscle group of the abdomen. The muscle group is used when flexing your ribcage toward your pelvis, and provides vital support to your midsection.

Position yourself lying flat on your back, with your knees bent and feet on the floor. Straighten your arms and rest your hands on the top of your thighs. Pull your chin in toward your chest very slightly so that your head lifts away from the floor. Breathe out and flatten your stomach as if pulling your belly button toward your lower back then squeeze the muscles so that they are tight. Hold this position throughout the exercise.

Reach your hands up your thighs and touch the top of your knees, curling your shoulders toward your pelvis, but not

lifting your lower back. Pause, and then slowly uncurl, sliding your hands back down your thighs until you are back to the start position, but not resting down completely. Focusing on a reference point on the ceiling will help you to fix your head and neck in position for the duration of the exercise.

Muscle group worked in this exercise: Abdomen (rectus abdominis).

Breathing tip: Breathe out as you reach to knees.

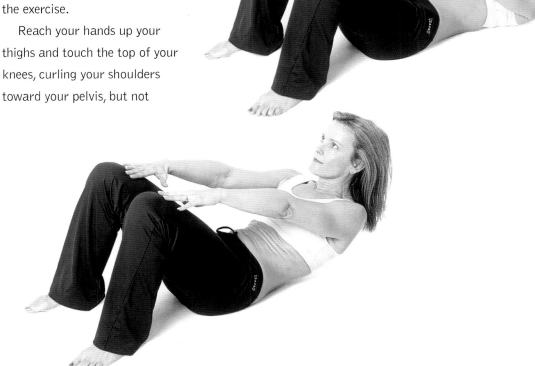

Abdominal Reverse Curl

Midsection

This is another abdominal exercise designed to work the major muscle group of the abdomen, with more emphasis on the lower portion. No resistance band is required for this exercise.

Position yourself lying flat on your back. Breathe out and flatten your stomach as if pulling your belly button toward your lower back, then squeeze the muscles so that they are tight. Raise your legs so that your thighs are at 90 degrees to the floor, with feet elevated. Rest your arms on either side of your body to aid stability.

Raise your legs and bring knees back toward your head; your buttocks should lift from the floor very slightly. Pause, and then slowly uncurl lowering your pelvis until your legs return to the start position. Focus on contracting your abdomen and not the movement of the legs. Keep your neck and shoulders relaxed and on the floor throughout the exercise.

Muscle group worked in this exercise: Abdomen (rectus abdominis).

Breathing tip: Breathe out as you raise your legs toward you.

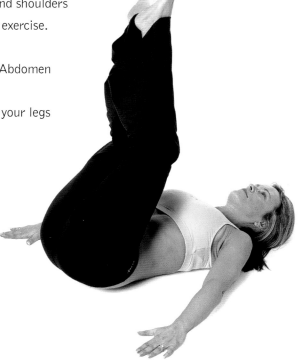

Abdominal Curl Twist
Midsection

This is a combination exercise designed to work the major muscle groups of the front and side of the abdomen. No resistance band is required.

Lie flat on your back, with thighs at 90-degrees to your body and feet elevated to knee height. Your arms should be bent with fingertips touching either side of your head. Pull your chin in toward your chest so head lifts away from the floor.

Lift your shoulders away from the floor and curl them toward your pelvis, rotating at the waist. Flex your hip on the opposite side bringing your knee toward the opposite elbow. Slowly uncurl and extend the hip until you are back to the start position with both thighs level.

Muscle groups worked in this exercise: Center of abdomen (rectus abdominis), external obliques.

Breathing tip: Breathe out as you reach elbow to knee.

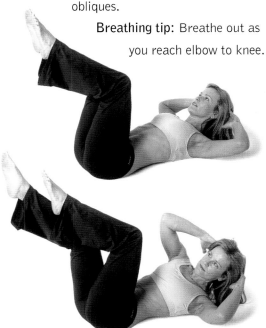

Dorsal Raises
Midsection

This is a basic yet effective exercise designed to work the major muscle group down the middle of your back, on either side of your spine. The muscle group, which is made up of four muscles, is worked when extending your back and provides vital support. No resistance band is required for this exercise.

Position yourself lying flat on your front with neck straight so that you are facing the floor. Legs should be straight and arms extended above your head.

Lift your left arm and right leg extending it at the hip, and keeping this arm and leg straight. Pause, and then slowly lower your arm and leg back down to the floor until you reach the start position. Then repeat with your right arm and left leg. Only lift as far as is comfortable. Your range of movement in the hip and shoulder should be increased progressively.

Muscle group worked in this exercise: Length of back (erector spinae).

Breathing tip: Breathe out as you lift opposite arm and leg.

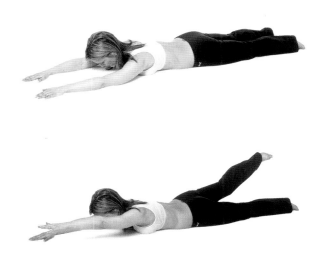

Kneeling Resisted Abdominal Curl

Midsection

This abdominal exercise is a progression from the standard Abdominal Curl. It is designed to work the major muscle group of the abdomen against a controlled resistance with more emphasis on the upper portion.

Attach the resistance band to a door anchor, or around a sturdy object of a suitable height, ensuring that it is positioned at least at head height when standing.

Position yourself kneeling down with the band in front of you. Take hold of the handles with a palms-in grip then place them on either side of your head. Lean forward so that your back is parallel to the floor, and with your buttocks elevated away from your heels. Breathe out and flatten your stomach as if pulling your belly button toward your lower back, then squeeze the muscles so that they are tight. Hold the contraction throughout the exercise.

Pull down against the resistance by rolling your shoulders toward your pelvis, and elbows to thighs. Pause and then slowly uncurl, raising the shoulders until you are back to the start position. Keep the angle in your hips and legs fixed throughout the exercise so that the target muscles are not being assisted.

Muscle group worked in this exercise: Abdomen (rectus abdominis).
Breathing tip: Breathe out as you roll shoulders toward your pelvis.

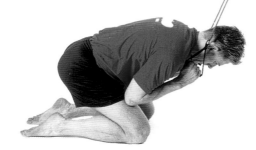

Side Bends

Midsection

This exercise is designed to work the muscles on either side of your midsection. They are worked in a lateral flexion (bending side to side) movement.

Attach the resistance band to a door anchor, or around a sturdy object ensuring that it is positioned at floor level. You only need to use one end of the band for this exercise, so ensure that the other end is securely attached to the anchor point.

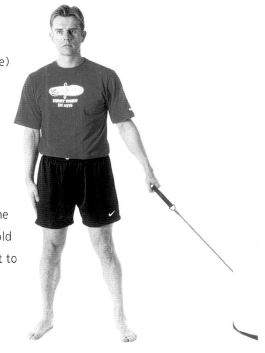

Position yourself with feet shoulder-width apart, and in the correct standing exercise posture. Keep abdominal muscles tight. The band should be coming from the side you are working on. Taking hold of the handle with an overhand grip, hold your arm straight and out to the side at a 45-degree angle to your body. There should be some resistance at this point.

Holding your lower body still and hips level, flex your midsection, leaning away from the anchor point and aiming to touch your free hand on the side of your knee. Pause, and then straighten your midsection back to the upright starting position. Turn around and repeat on your other side. Ensure that you don't sway your hips during the exercise. To make the exercise harder, step further away from the anchor point or make it easier by moving closer.

Muscle group worked in this exercise: Sides of midsection (external obliques).

Breathing tip: Breathe out as you laterally flex away from the anchor point.

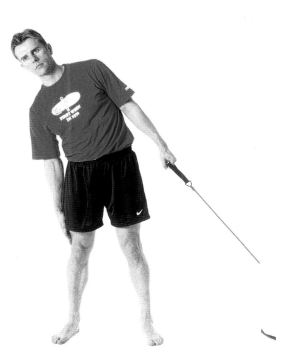

Resistance Band 30 Minute Workout

The 30 Minute Workout has been designed so that it is suitable for everyone, whether you're new to resistance training and want an effective and achievable starting point, or if you have time constraints and need a time-efficient workout. It includes all the major muscle groups and multi-joint exercises to ensure that the whole body has been worked, and because the workout has been formulated with time efficiency in mind, idle periods, such as resting time between sets, have been utilized for flexibility exercises, saving you valuable time and enabling you to get more from your workout.

Exercise Format Example: Having warmed up, start the first exercise, Chest Press. Complete your first set of 12–15 repetitions (using it to progressively increase the exercise intensity and range of movement). Hold the Chest Stretch flexibility exercise for 15 seconds, then complete your final set of 12–15 Chest Press repetitions. Reposition the equipment for the next exercise and start its first set. Continue in this format until you have completed all the exercises in this workout.

Warm Up

A pre-resistance band warm-up should be performed for at least 10 minutes and should focus on all areas of the body. As the 30 Minute Workout was designed to suit people with a small amount of training time, the full workout has been condensed to add flexibility exercises into the program, making it more achievable, beneficial, and safe.

Here are some simple, yet effective, aerobic exercises that you can use in your pre-resistance band workout warm-up program in any environment. You can start by doing one minute of each.

The warm-up exercises can also be used at the end of your workout as a cool-down phase, with very light aerobic movements to reduce heart rate.

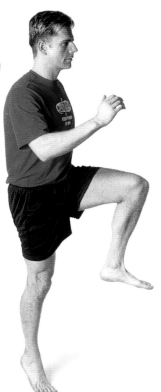

Jogging on the Spot

Gentle jogging is a great way of warming up, as you are using the large muscle groups in your legs and controlling your body weight. You can do this on the spot, or moving forward as if in an open area. To get the most from this exercise as a warm-up, progressively raise knees higher and use large opposite arm and leg movements, lifting hands to head level.

Star Jumps

Star jumps are good for warming up areas that are not used much in jogging, because you are moving your limbs out to the side and back in, rather than forward and backward, as in jogging. Therefore areas such as the middle and the top of the shoulder and the outer and inner thigh are being prepared.

Start by standing straight with feet together and arms by your side. Jump feet out, landing in a wide stance, and simultaneously lift arms out to the side and above your head, keeping them straight. As soon as your feet touch the floor, jump back to the start position. Continue to repeat this movement.

Shadow Punch / Leg Strides

This warm-up exercise is great as it allows you to progressively work the chest, arms, shoulders, and upper back, as well as legs, hips, and midsection through slight rotation. This also helps you to develop cross-body coordination by using an opposite arm and leg movement.

Start with one arm forward with the palm of your hand facing down and in a fist, and the opposite leg forward. The other arm should be bent and close to your body, with the palm of your hand facing up with a clenched fist, and opposite leg back. Keeping the weight on your toes, jump, swapping your leg position in one large stride. Simultaneously punch your other arm forward and bring the extended one back. Once your toes have made contact with the ground, jump back to the start position and continue to repeat.

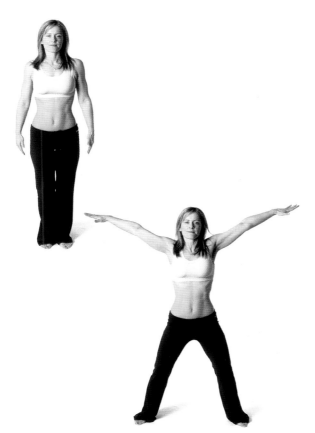

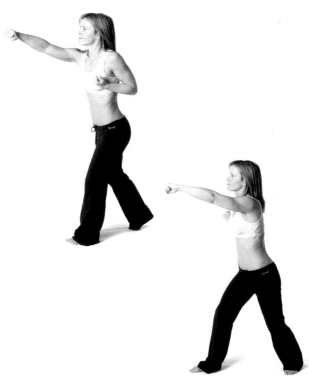

Chest Press

Sets: 2 / Repetitions: 12–15

Direction of resistance: From behind

Hold the handles of the band in each hand with an overhand grip and elbows bent at 90 degrees. Ensure that elbows and wrists are all elevated to shoulder height and are parallel to the floor.

Extend both arms forward until they are straight, and then slowly bend arms back to the start position, stopping when you feel a slight stretch across your chest and shoulders. To make the exercise harder, step further forward, or make it easier by moving closer to the attachment.

Muscle groups worked in this exercise: Chest (pectorals), front of shoulders (anterior deltoid), and back of upper arms (triceps).

Breathing tip: Breathe out as you extend arms forward.

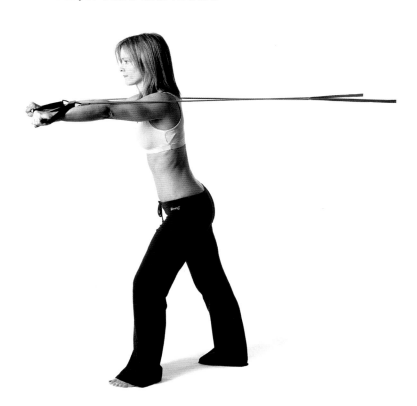

Stretch between sets: Chest

Bend elbows to 90 degrees and raise your arms out to
the side with hands in the air, until elbows are at
shoulder height. Pull elbows back, retracting your
shoulders and sticking out your chest until you feel a
stretch across your chest and in the front of your
shoulders. Hold the stretch for 15 seconds.

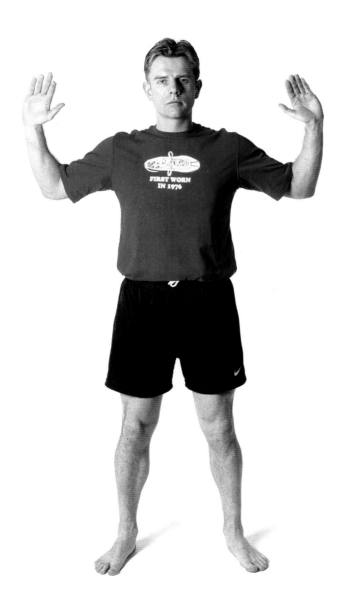

Latissimus Pull Down

Sets: 2 / Repetitions: 12–15

Direction of resistance: From above/in front

Hold the handles of the band in each hand with palms facing forward and arms extended toward the anchor point.

Pull the band down in a straight line by bending arms, keeping a wide-arm position, until your elbows pass the line of your back and reach your sides. You should feel a slight stretch across your chest—if not, ensure that you are squeezing your shoulder blades together at the bottom of the movement. Then extend your arms following the same line, until they are back to the start position. At this point they should be fully extended before beginning your next repetition.

Muscle groups worked in this exercise: Back (latissimus dorsi), back of shoulders (posterior deltoid), and front of upper arms (biceps).

Breathing tip: Breathe out as you pull down.

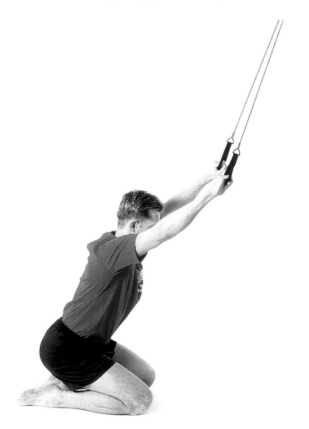
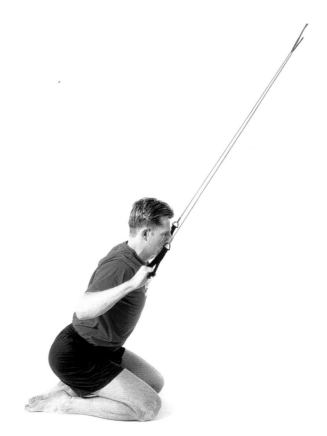

Stretch between sets: Combined Upper Body Stretch

Kneel down with arms extended. Lower your head between your shoulders and then slowly sit down onto your heels, pulling back against your hands.

Slowly walk both hands around, reaching to one side, so that you are flexing laterally at the waist. Hold this position for 15 seconds, then walk your hands back to the center and repeat on the other side, holding the stretch again for 15 seconds.

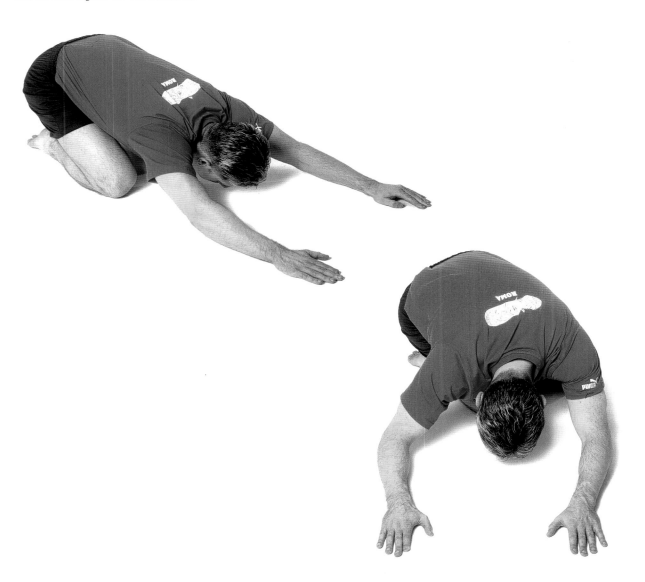

Shoulder Press

Sets: 2 / Repetitions: 12–15

Direction of resistance: From underneath

Sit up straight with shoulders back and abdominal muscles tight. Using an overhand grip hold the handles at the side of each shoulder, and at shoulder height.

Extend both arms above your head until they are straight and then slowly bend arms, taking them back to the start position, with your hands returning level with shoulders. Make sure that your forearms remain vertical throughout the movement.

Muscle groups worked in this exercise: Front of shoulders (anterior deltoid), top of shoulders (upper trapezius), and back of upper arms (triceps).

Breathing tip: Breathe out as you extend arms up.

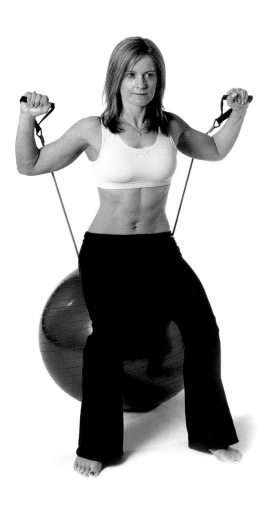

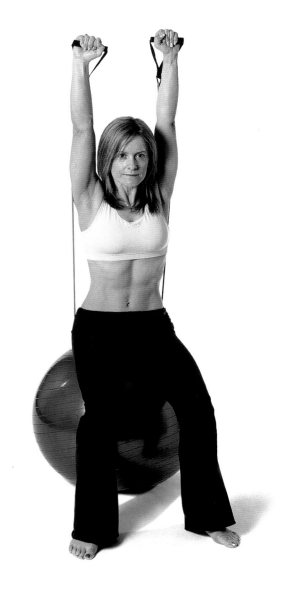

Stretch between sets: Triceps

Stand straight. Raise one arm up above your head, bend it at the elbow and place your hand behind you, touching between your shoulder blades. Lift the other arm above your head and cup your hand just above the elbow of the first arm. Ease the first arm back until you feel the stretch in the back of the upper arm. Hold this stretch for 15 seconds and then repeat with your other arm.

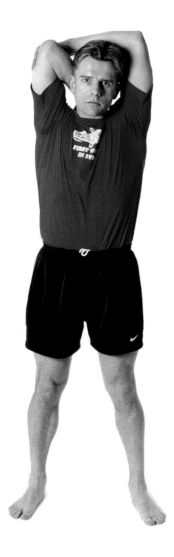

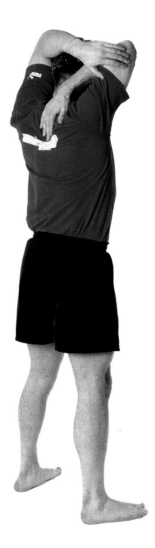

Squat

Sets: 2 / Repetitions: 12–15

Direction of resistance: From underneath

Place band under both feet and position them shoulder-width apart. Take hold of the handles with an overhand grip at shoulder level with the palm of your hands facing forward.

Slowly bend your knees, keeping your heels down, as if you were about to sit down, stopping just before you reach a 90-degree angle. Pause, then extend your legs, pushing through your heels until you are back to the starting position. You can keep feet wider apart to make the exercise harder or closer to make it easier.

Muscle groups worked in this exercise: Front of thigh (quadriceps), buttocks (gluteus maximus).

Breathing tip: Breathe out as you extend legs.

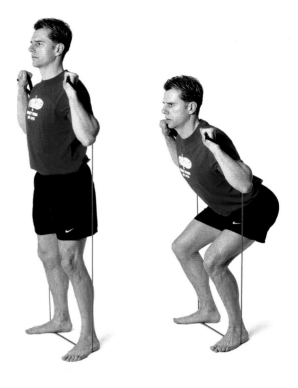

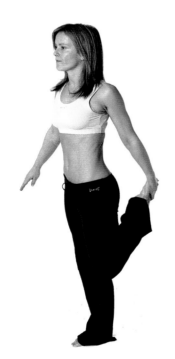

Stretch between sets: Quadriceps

Stand on your right leg. Bend the knee of your left leg and take hold of your ankle with your left arm, lifting it up behind you, so that your heel is near to your buttocks. Make sure that your body is completely straight with hips forward, legs close together, and knees in line. Hold the stretch for 15 seconds and then repeat with your right leg.

Standing Hamstring Curl

Sets: 2 / Repetitions: 12–15

Direction of resistance: From front

Attach one end of the band to an ankle strap and then place around the ankle of the leg that you are starting with. You can place a stable object next to you to hold onto for support.

Flex one leg at the knee until the lower leg is at 90 degrees to the upper. Pause, and then extend the leg at the knee until your leg is straight. Ensure that your hips remain still and keep both knees together throughout the exercise. Repeat using your other leg. To make the exercise harder, step further away from the anchor point, or make it easier by moving closer.

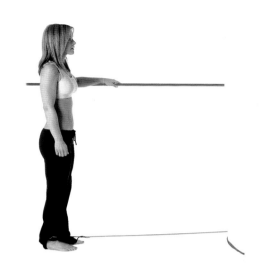

Muscle groups worked in this exercise: Back of upper leg (hamstrings).

Breathing tip: Breathe out as you bend the knee.

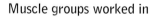

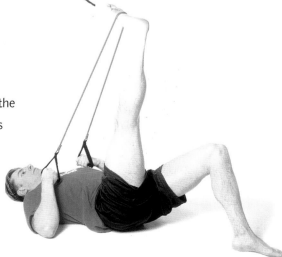

Stretch between sets: Lying Hamstrings

Bend one leg at the knee with your foot on the floor. Place the band over the foot of the other leg and extend it so that it is straight. Keeping your lower back and buttocks flat on the floor, flex the hip of the straight leg, bringing your thigh back as far as possible without bending at the knee. Use the band to aid and progressively increase the stretch. Hold the stretch for 15 seconds and then repeat with the other leg.

Abdominal Curl

Sets: 2 / Repetitions: 12–15

Direction of resistance: No band required

Lie flat on your back, with your knees bent and feet on the floor. Breathe out and flatten your stomach, as if pulling your belly button toward your lower back, then squeeze the muscles so that they are tight. Hold this position throughout the exercise.

Reach hands up your thighs and touch the top of your knees, curling your shoulders toward your pelvis. Pause, and then slowly uncurl, sliding your hands back down your thighs until you are back to the start position.

Muscle group worked in this exercise: Abdomen (rectus abdominis).

Breathing tip: Breathe out as you reach to knees.

Stretch between sets: Lie Flat

Rest between sets of Abdominal Curls by lying completely flat on your back, with legs stretched out straight and arms extended and touching the floor above your head. Hold this position for 20 seconds.

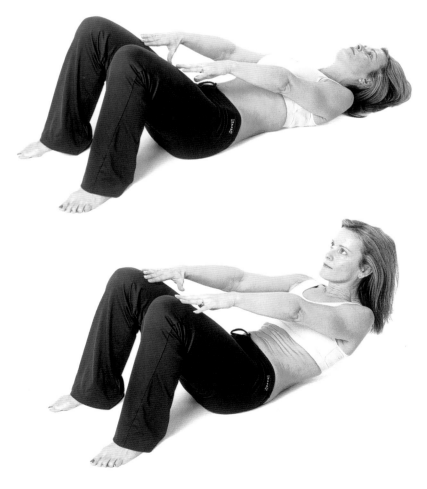

Dorsal Raises

Sets: 2 / Repetitions: 12–15

Direction of resistance: No band required

Lie flat on your front with head straight. Legs should be straight and arms extended above your head.

Lift your left arm and right leg, extending it at the hip and keeping both arm and leg straight. Pause, and then slowly lower your arm and leg back down to the floor until you reach the start position. Then repeat with your right arm and left leg.

Muscle group worked in this exercise: Length of back (erector spinae).

Breathing tip: Breathe out as you lift opposite arm and leg.

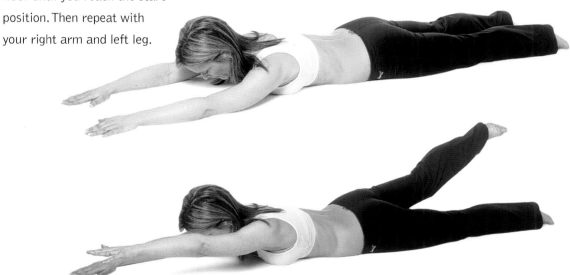

Stretch between sets: Lower Back

Lie on your back; bend your knees, bringing them up toward your chest. Place your arms behind your knees and gently pull them in close to your body. You can increase the area of the stretch by rolling your shoulders forward and tucking your head in. Hold the stretch for at least 15 seconds.

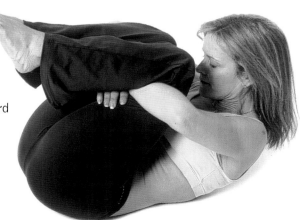

Resistance Band 60 Minute Workout

The 60 Minute Workout has been designed as a progression from the 30-minute version. If you are new to resistance training, it would be advisable to start with the 30 Minute Workout and then build up to the longer routine. Rest time between sets has been utilized for flexibility exercises, enabling you to get more benefit from the workout time. This also gives you a better understanding of which areas you should be stretching when developing your own program.

Exercise Format Example: Having warmed up, start the first exercise, Chest Press. Complete your first set of 12–15 repetitions (using it to progressively increase the exercise intensity and range of movement). Hold the Chest Stretch flexibility exercise for 15 seconds, then complete your final set of 12–15 Chest Press repetitions. Reposition the equipment for the next exercise and start its first set. Continue in this format until you have completed all the exercises in this workout.

Warm Up

Before exercising, a warm-up should be performed for at least 10 minutes and should focus on all areas of the body. Here are some simple, yet effective, aerobic exercises that you can incorporate into your pre-resistance band workout warm-up program, in any situation. Start by doing two minutes of each.

The following warm-up exercises can also be used at the end of your workout as a cool-down phase, with very light aerobic movements to reduce heart rate.

Jogging on the Spot

Gentle jogging is a great way of warming up as you are using the large muscle groups in your legs and controlling your body weight. You can do this on the spot, or moving forward, as if in an open area. To get the most from this exercise as a warm-up, progressively raise your knees higher and use large opposite arm and leg movements, lifting hands to head level.

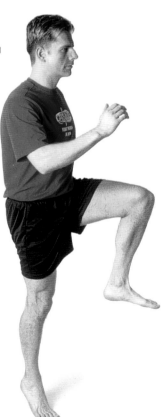

Star Jumps

Star jumps are good for warming up areas that are not used much in jogging, because you are moving your limbs out to the side and back in, rather than forward and backward in jogging. Therefore areas such as the middle and the top of the shoulder, and the outer and inner thigh, are being prepared.

Start by standing straight with feet together and arms by your side. Jump feet out, landing in a wide stance, and simultaneously lift arms out to the side and above your head, keeping them straight. As soon as your feet touch the floor, jump back to the start position. Continue to repeat this movement.

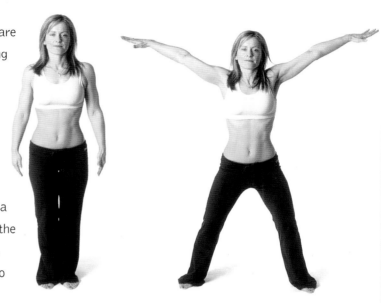

Shadow Punches / Leg Strides

This warm-up exercise is great as it allows you to progressively work the chest, arms, shoulders, and upper back, as well as legs, hips, and midsection through slight rotation. This also helps you to develop cross-body coordination by using an opposite arm and leg movement.

Start with one arm forward with the palm of your hand facing down and in a fist, and the opposite leg forward. The other arm should be bent and close to your body, with the palm of your hand facing up with a clenched fist, and opposite leg back. Keeping the weight on your toes, jump, swapping your leg position in one large stride. Simultaneously punch your other arm forward and bring the extended one back. Once your toes have made contact with the ground, jump back to the start position and continue to repeat.

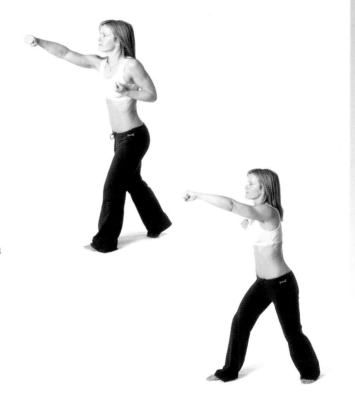

Chest Press

Sets: 2 / Repetitions: 12–15

Direction of resistance: From behind

Hold the handles of the band in each hand with an overhand grip and elbows bent at 90 degrees. Ensure that elbows and wrists are all elevated to shoulder height and are parallel to the floor.

Extend both arms forward until they are straight, and then slowly bend arms back to the start position, stopping when you feel a slight stretch across your chest and shoulders. To make the exercise harder, step further forward, or make it easier by moving closer to the attachment.

Muscle groups worked in this exercise: Chest (pectorals), front of shoulders (anterior deltoid), and back of upper arms (triceps).

Breathing tip: Breathe out as you extend arms forward.

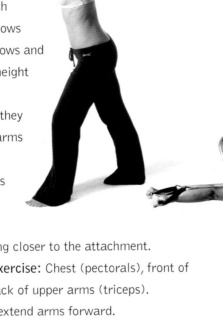

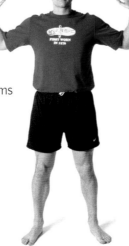

Stretch between sets: Chest

Bend elbows to 90 degrees and raise your arms out to the side with hands in the air, until elbows are at shoulder height. Pull elbows back, retracting your shoulders and sticking out your chest until you feel a stretch across your chest and in the front of your shoulders. Hold the stretch for 15 seconds.

Standing Mid Row

Sets: 2 / Repetitions: 12–15

Direction of resistance: From front

Hold the handles of the band with palms facing down and arms extended forward until they are straight. Elbows and wrists should be elevated to shoulder height and parallel to the floor.

Slowly bend elbows, pulling them back past the line of your shoulders, ensuring that elbows and wrists remain elevated to shoulder height and parallel to the floor. Then slowly straighten your arms back to the start position, stopping when they are fully extended. To make the exercise harder, step further back, or make it easier by moving closer to the attachment.

Muscle groups worked in this exercise: Upper back (lower trapezius), back of shoulders (posterior deltoid), between shoulders (rhomboids), and front of upper arms (biceps).

Breathing tip: Breathe out as you pull arms backward.

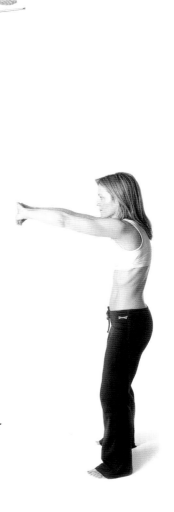

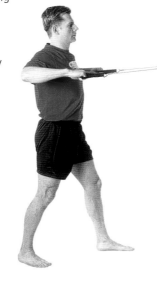

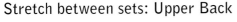

Stretch between sets: Upper Back

Stand with feet hip-width apart and knees slightly bent. Interlock fingers and rotate your wrists so that your palms are facing forward. Extend your arms, pushing your hands forward until your arms are straight. Round your shoulders to protract the shoulder blades and tilt your pelvis back very slightly. Hold the stretch for 15 seconds.

Upright Row

Sets: 2 / Repetitions: 12–15

Direction of resistance: From below

With the resistance band under the arches of both feet, place them hip-width apart and swap the handles of the band to opposite hands so that it crosses over, holding them with a close overhand grip. Extend arms down toward the floor until they are straight, but don't round your shoulders.

With elbows leading, lift the handles of the band until your hands reach your chin, keeping them close to your body throughout the movement. Then return back to the start position, stopping when they are fully extended. Ensure that your back remains still throughout the exercise. You can move feet wider apart to make the exercise harder, or closer to make it easier.

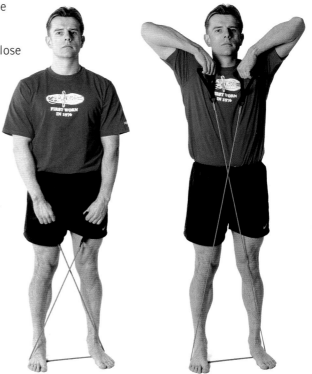

Muscle groups worked in this exercise: Upper back/neck (upper and lower trapezius), front and middle of shoulder (anterior and medial deltoid), and front of upper arms (biceps).

Breathing tip: Breathe out as you pull arms up.

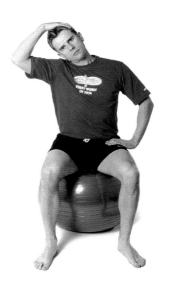

Stretch between sets: Neck Lateral Flexion

Sit down with your shoulders back and abdominal muscle tight to avoid slouching. Lower your ear toward the shoulder of the same side, until you feel a stretch in the neck and shoulder of the opposite side. You can control and increase the stretch by placing your hand over your head and easing it a little further. Hold the stretch for 15 second and then repeat on the other side.

Tricep Extension

Sets: 2 / Repetitions: 12–15
Direction of Resistance: From above /in front
Position yourself so that the band is as vertical as possible, with feet hip-width apart and in the correct standing exercise posture. Take hold of the handles with an overhand grip and with elbows locked in by your sides. Bend your arms until hands are at shoulder height.

Extend your arms, pushing the handles down until they touch your thighs. Pause, and then bend your arms, returning your hands back to the start position. Ensure that you keep your upper arm and elbows fixed by your sides and do not let them spring out.

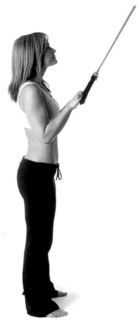
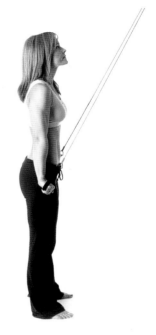

Muscle group worked in this exercise: Back of upper arms (triceps).
Breathing tip: Breathe out as you straighten arms.

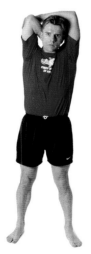
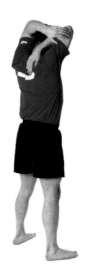

Stretch between sets: Triceps

Raise one arm up above your head, bend it at the elbow and place your hand behind you, touching between your shoulder blades. Lift the other arm above your head and cup your hand just above the elbow of your first arm. Ease the first arm back until you feel the stretch in the back of the upper arm. Hold this stretch for 15 seconds and then repeat with your other arm.

Bicep Curls

Sets: 2 / Repetitions: 12–15

Direction of resistance: From below

Place the resistance band under the arches of both feet. Position yourself with feet hip-width apart and in the correct standing exercise posture. Take hold of the handles with an underhand grip and arms straight by your side.

Lift your hands in front of you by flexing at the elbow, keeping a strict position with the upper arms locked by your sides. Pause when your hands are at chest height, but not touching, and then slowly straighten arms back to the starting position, stopping when your hands reach the side of your legs. To make the exercise harder, move feet further apart, or make it easier by moving them closer together.

Muscle group worked in this exercise: Front of upper arms (biceps).

Breathing tip: Breathe out as you bring your hands up.

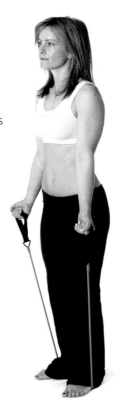
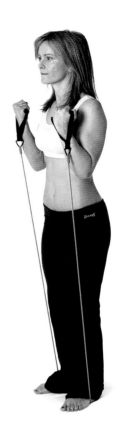

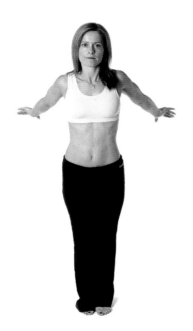

Stretch between sets: Biceps

Position yourself with feet shoulder-width apart and body straight. Elevate both arms out to the side of your body and pull them back. Rotate your wrists inward until your palms are facing up and you feel a stretch in your biceps and upper forearm. Hold the stretch for 15 seconds.

Hip / Leg Extension

Sets: 2 / Repetitions: 12–15

Direction of resistance: From above the hip

Position yourself on your hands and knees, or elbows if it is more comfortable. Place the resistance band in the arch of one of your feet. Take hold of both handles with a palms-in grip and with the band on the inside of your arms. Raise the knee of the side you are working toward your chest.

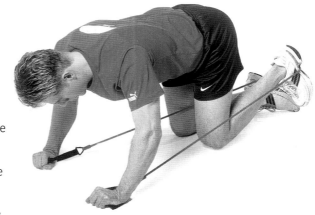

Extend your hip and leg. Push your foot directly behind you, stopping when it forms a straight line with your body and your foot is at hip height. Pause, and then flex your hip and bend your knee, bringing it back toward your chest and to the start position. Repeat on your other side.

Muscle group worked in this exercise: Buttocks (gluteus maximus).
Breathing tip: Breathe out as you extend hip leg.

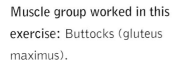

Stretch between sets: Gluteus — Knee to Chest

Lie down on the floor with one leg straight. Bend the knee of your other leg and bring it in toward your chest. Place your hands behind your knee and pull in toward you. Make sure that your neck and shoulders are relaxed. Hold the stretch for 15 seconds and then repeat on the other side.

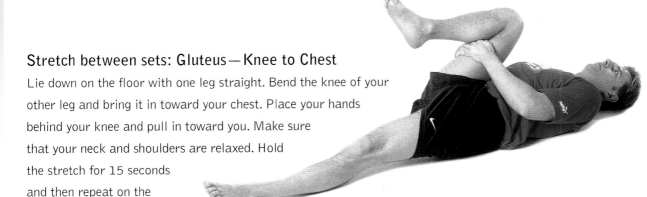

Standing Leg Extension

Sets: 2 / Repetitions: 12–15

Direction of resistance: From behind

Position yourself so that the band is coming from behind you and make sure you are in the correct standing posture. Stand on one leg, flexing the other at the hip so that the thigh is at 45 degrees. Bend the knee of the elevated leg so that your foot drops back. Place a stable object next to you for support.

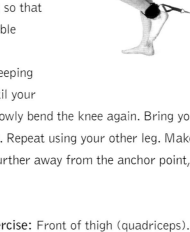

Extend your leg at the knee, keeping the upper part of the leg still, until your leg is straight. Pause, and then slowly bend the knee again. Bring your foot back to the starting position. Repeat using your other leg. Make the exercise harder by stepping further away from the anchor point, or make it easier by moving closer.

Muscle group worked in this exercise: Front of thigh (quadriceps).
Breathing tip: Breathe out as you extend leg.

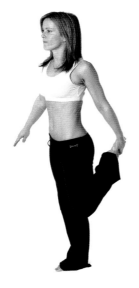

Stretch between sets: Quadriceps

Stand on your right leg. Bend the knee of your left leg and take hold of your ankle with your left arm, lifting it up behind you, so that your heel is near to your buttocks. Make sure that your body is straight with hips forward, legs close together, and knees in line. Hold the stretch for 15 seconds and then repeat with your right leg.

Lying Hamstring Curl

Sets: 2 / Repetitions: 12–15

Direction of resistance: From behind the feet

Position yourself lying on your front. Attach the ankle strap to one ankle, with the band coming from behind your feet and both legs straight.

Bend the knee of the leg you're exercising until your heel is near to your buttocks. Pause, and then slowly extend your leg again. Straighten the leg and bring it back to the starting position. Repeat using your other leg. Ensure that your hips remain still and keep knees together throughout the exercise.

Muscle group worked in this exercise: Back of upper leg (hamstrings).

Breathing tip: Breathe out as you bend the knee.

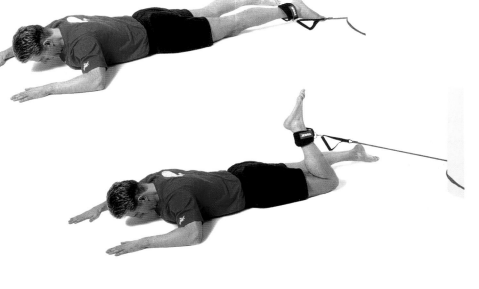

Stretch between sets: Lying Hamstrings

Bend one leg at the knee with foot on the floor. Place the band over the foot of the other and extend it so that it is straight. Keeping your lower back and buttocks flat on the floor, flex the hip of the straight leg, bringing your thigh back as far as possible without bending at the knee. Use the band to aid and progressively increase the stretch. Hold the stretch for 15 seconds and then repeat with the other leg.

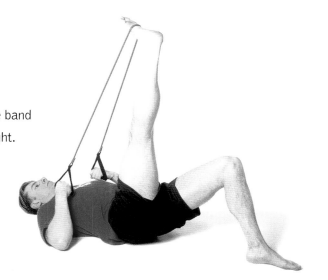

Standing Outer Thigh

Sets: 2 / Repetitions: 12–15

Direction of resistance: From the side

Attach the band to an ankle strap,
placing it around the ankle of the leg
that you are working. Stand side-on to
the anchor point, with the band attached
to the leg that is furthest away. The leg
that you are working should cross over the
front of the other. Have a stable object next
to you for support.

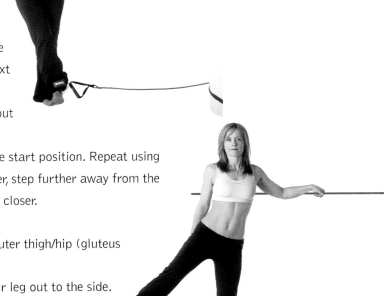

Lift (abduct) the leg you are working out
to the side to a 40- to 45-degree angle.
Pause, and then lower your leg back to the start position. Repeat using
your other leg. To make the exercise harder, step further away from the
anchor point, or make it easier by moving closer.

Muscle group worked in this exercise: Outer thigh/hip (gluteus
medius).

Breathing tip: Breathe out as you lift your leg out to the side.

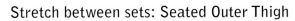

Stretch between sets: Seated Outer Thigh

Sit with your right leg straight. Bend your left leg and place your foot
over the outside of your right knee. Reach your left arm behind you and
rotate your shoulders to the left so that they are parallel to your
legs. Extend your right arm, placing it across the
outside of your left leg and gently ease it across
to the right. Hold the stretch for 15 seconds,
and then repeat with the opposite side.

Calf Flex

Sets: 2 / Repetitions: 12–15

Direction of resistance: From above the foot

Place both resistance band handles around the ball of
one foot. Take hold of the middle of the band with an
overhand grip, and bring hands up to chest level.
Extend the leg with the band attached, so that it
is straight and off the ground.

Push your toes down against the band, pivoting
at the ankle, as if pushing on a brake pedal.
Pause, and then lift your toes back as far as
possible, to the start position. Repeat with the
other leg. You can move hands wider apart to
make the exercise harder, or closer to make it
easier.

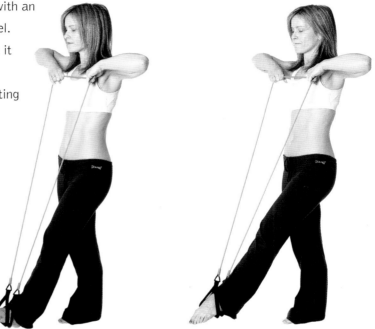

Muscle group worked in this exercise:
Back of lower leg (calf).
Breathing tip: Breathe out as you
push toes down.

Stretch between sets: Gastrocnemius

Stand about a foot (30cms) away from a wall or
another sturdy object. Lean in and place your hands
against the wall for support. Take a large step back
with one leg, keeping it straight. Slowly bend the knee
of the leading leg until you feel a stretch in the back
and bottom of the straightened leg. Keep heels down
throughout the stretch. Hold for 15 seconds and then
repeat with your other leg.

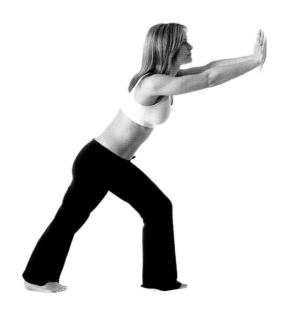

Abdominal Curl Twist

Sets: 2 / Repetitions: 12–15

Direction of resistance: No band required

Lie on your back, with your thighs at 90 degrees to your body and feet elevated to knee height. Touch fingertips to either side of your head. Breathe out and flatten your stomach as if pulling your belly button toward your lower back, then squeeze the muscles so that they are tight. Hold the contraction throughout the exercise.

Lift and curl your shoulders toward your pelvis, rotating at the waist. Simultaneously flex your hip on the opposite side, bringing your knee toward the opposite elbow. Pause, and then slowly uncurl and extend the hip until you are back to the start position with both thighs level. Continue to repeat on the opposite side.

Muscle groups worked in this exercise: Center of abdomen (rectus abdominis), either side of abdomen (external obliques).

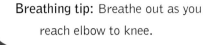

Breathing tip: Breathe out as you reach elbow to knee.

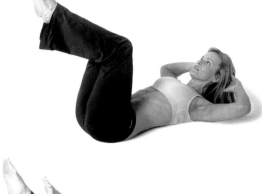

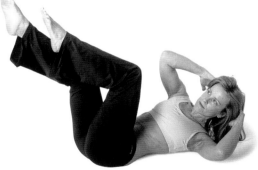

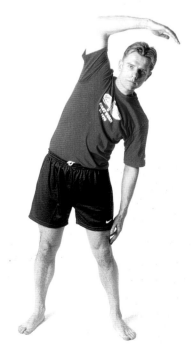

Stretch between sets: Sides

Lift one arm up, raising your hand as high as possible, then laterally flex at the waist, reaching your arm over and across in the same direction until you feel the stretch in your side. Hold this position for 15 seconds and then repeat on the other side. Make sure that you don't lean forward or backward during the stretch. You can also try this seated.

Dorsal Raises

Sets: 2 / Repetitions: 12–15

Direction of resistance: No band required

Lie flat on your front with head straight. Legs should be straight and arms extended above your head.

Lift your left arm and right leg, extending it at the hip and keeping both arm and leg straight. Pause, and then slowly lower your arm and leg back down to the floor until you reach the start position. Then repeat with your right arm and left leg.

Muscle group worked in this exercise: Length of back (erector spinae).

Breathing tip: Breathe out as you lift opposite arm and leg.

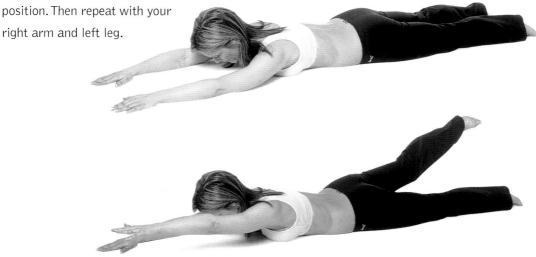

Stretch between sets: Lower Back

Lie on your back; bend your knees bringing them up toward your chest. Place your arms behind your knees and gently pull them in close to your body. You can increase the area of the stretch by rolling your shoulders forward and tucking your head in. Hold the stretch for at least 15 seconds.

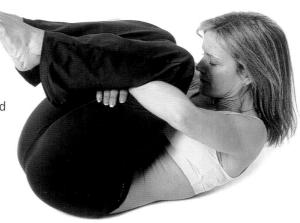

Resistance Band Skiing Workout

There are many reasons why people should carry out resistance training prior to going skiing. The most obvious reason is not to ruin a great vacation by experiencing the onset of muscle soreness and fatigue after the first day on the slopes. Resistance training will enable you to prepare your muscles for the event, allowing you to enjoy it to the full, while helping prevent injury at the same time.

Ensure that you warm up for at least 10 minutes prior to starting the workout (see page 72).

Squat

Sets: 2 / Repetitions: 12–15

Direction of resistance: From under foot

Place band under both feet and position them shoulder width apart. Take hold of the handles with an overhand grip at shoulder level with the palm of your hands facing forward.

Slowly bend your knees, keeping your heels down, as if you were about to sit down, stopping just before you reach a 90-degree angle. Pause, and then extend your legs, pushing through your heels until you are back to the starting position. You can move feet wider apart to make the exercise harder, or closer to make it easier.

Muscle groups worked in this exercise: Front of thigh (quadriceps), buttocks (gluteus maximus).

Breathing Tip: Breathe out as you extend legs.

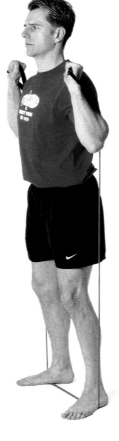
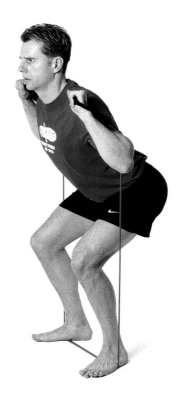

Lunge

Sets: 2 / Repetitions: 12–15

Direction of resistance: From under foot

From standing, take a large step forward with one foot and place the band underneath it. Keep both legs extended, feet parallel, with your leading foot flat and the heel of your back foot raised. Hold the handles of the band with an overhand grip and bring them up to shoulder level with the palms of your hands facing forward.

Bend your knees, stopping just before the knee of your back leg touches the floor, and both legs are bent to a 90-degree angle. Pause, and then extend your legs, pushing through the heel of the leading leg until you are back to the start position. Try to keep your back as vertical as possible throughout the exercise. Ensure that the knee of your leading leg remains in line with your ankle as your knee bends.

Muscle groups worked in this exercise: Front of thigh (quadriceps), buttocks (gluteus maximus).
Breathing tip: Breathe out as you extend legs.

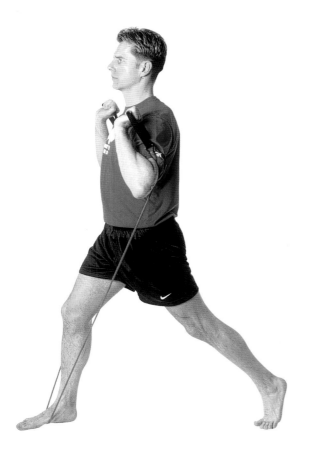
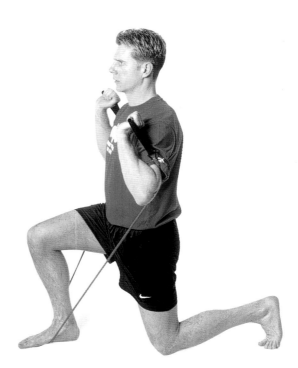

Hip Flexion

Sets: 2 / Repetitions: 12–15

Direction of resistance: From behind

Attach the band to an ankle strap then place it around the ankle of the leg that you are starting with. Position yourself so that the band is coming from behind you. Stand on one leg, extending the other at the hip and knee so that the thigh is at 30 degrees behind you. Keep your body upright and abdominal muscles tight. You can place a stable object next to you for support.

In a forward movement, flex your hip, allow the knee to bend, and lift knee as high as possible toward your chest without moving your back out of the upright position. Pause, and then slowly lower your knee, extending your hip and leg back to the starting position. Repeat using your other leg. Ensure that your upper body remains still throughout the exercise. To make the exercise harder, step further away from the anchor point, or make it easier by moving closer.

Muscle group worked in this exercise: Hip flexors (iliopsoas).

Breathing tip: Breathe out as you lift knee.

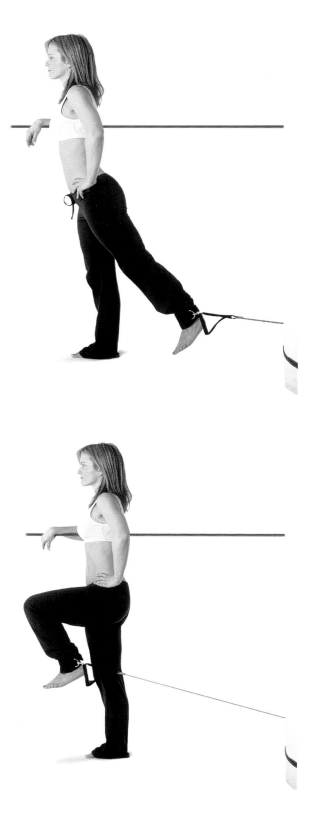

Lying Hamstring Curl

Sets: 2 / Repetitions: 12–15

Direction of resistance: From behind

Attach one end of the band to an ankle strap and then place around the ankle of the leg that you are starting with. Position yourself lying on your front, with the band coming from behind your feet and both legs straight.

Bend the knee of the leg you're exercising until your heel is near to your buttocks. Pause, and then slowly extend your leg again. Straighten it and bring it back to the starting position. Repeat using your other leg. Ensure that your hips remain still and keep your knees together throughout the exercise.

Muscle group worked in this exercise: Back of upper leg (hamstrings).

Breathing tip: Breathe out as you bend the knee.

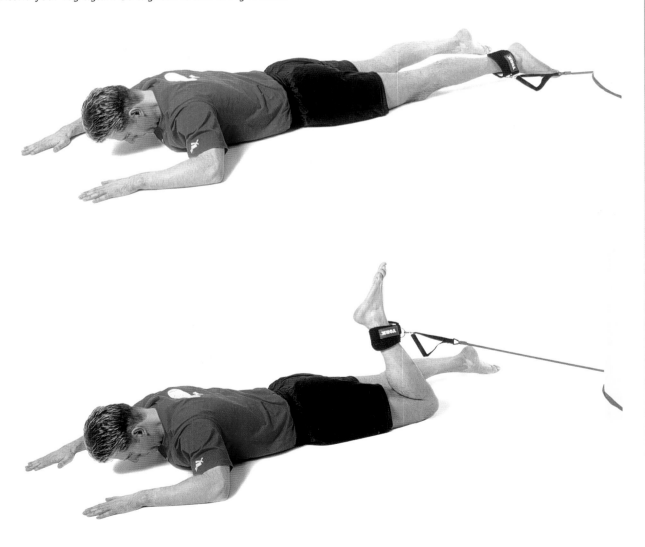

Latissimus Pull Down

Sets: 2 / Repetitions: 12–15

Direction of resistance: From above/in front

Hold the handles of the band in each hand with palms facing forward and arms extended toward the anchor point.

Pull the band down in a straight line by bending arms, keeping a wide-arm position, until your elbows pass the line of your back and reach your sides. You should feel a slight stretch across your chest—if not, ensure that you are squeezing your shoulder blades together at the bottom of the movement. Then extend your arms following the same line, until they are back to the start position. At this point they should be fully extended before beginning your next repetition.

Muscle groups worked in this exercise: Back (latissimus dorsi), back of shoulders (posterior deltoid), and front of upper arms (biceps).

Breathing tip: Breathe out as you pull down.

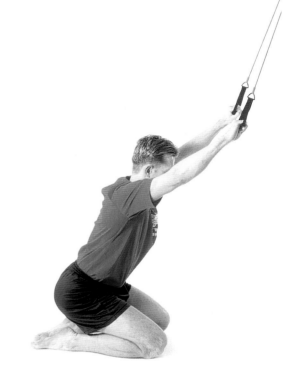

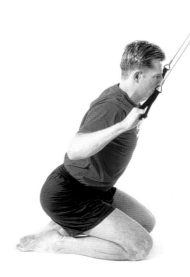

Chest Press

Sets: 2 / Repetitions: 12–15

Direction of resistance: From behind

Hold the handles of the band in each hand with an overhand grip and elbows bent at 90 degrees. Ensure that elbows and wrists are all elevated to shoulder height and are parallel to the floor.

Extend both arms forward until they are straight and then slowly bend arms back to the start position, stopping when you feel a slight stretch across your chest and shoulders. To make the exercise harder, step further forward, or make it easier by moving closer to the attachment.

Muscle groups worked in this exercise: Chest (pectorals), front of shoulders (anterior deltoid), and back of upper arms (triceps).

Breathing tip: Breathe out as you extend arms forward.

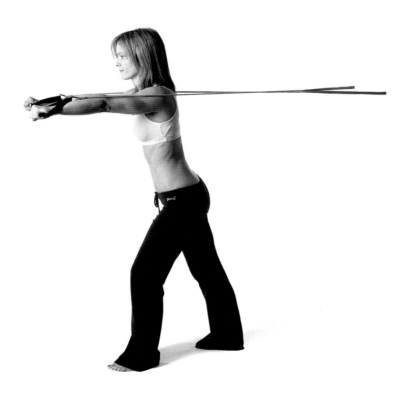

Shoulder Press

Sets: 2 / Repetitions: 12–15

Direction of resistance: From underneath

Sit up straight with shoulders back and abdominal muscles tight. Using an overhand grip hold the handles at the side of each shoulder and at shoulder height.

Extend both arms above your head until they are straight and then slowly bend arms, taking them back to the start position, with your hands returning level with your shoulders. Make sure that your forearms remain vertical throughout the movement.

Muscle groups worked in this exercise: Front of shoulders (anterior deltoid), top of shoulders (upper trapezius), and back of upper arms (triceps).

Breathing tip: Breathe out as you extend arms up.

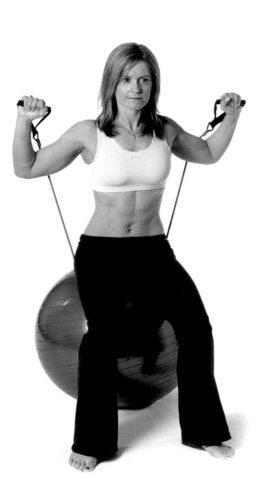

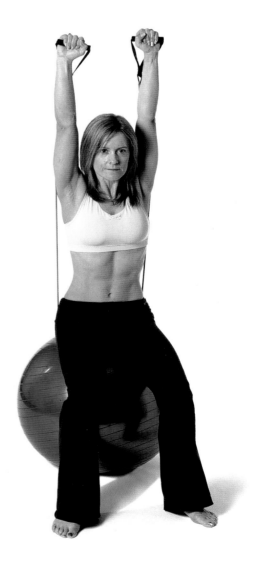

Standing Outer Thigh

Sets: 2 / Repetitions: 12–15

Direction of resistance: From the far side

Attach the band to an ankle strap, placing it around the ankle of the leg that you are working. Stand side-on to the anchor point, with the band attached to the leg that is furthest away. The leg that you are working should cross over the front of the other. Have a stable object next to you for support.

Lift (abduct) the leg you are working out to the side to a 40- to 45-degree angle. Pause, and then lower your leg back to the start position. Repeat using your other leg. To make the exercise harder, step further away from the anchor point, or make it easier by moving closer.

Muscle groups worked in this exercise: Outer thigh/hip (gluteus medius).

Breathing tip: Breathe out as you lift leg out to the side.

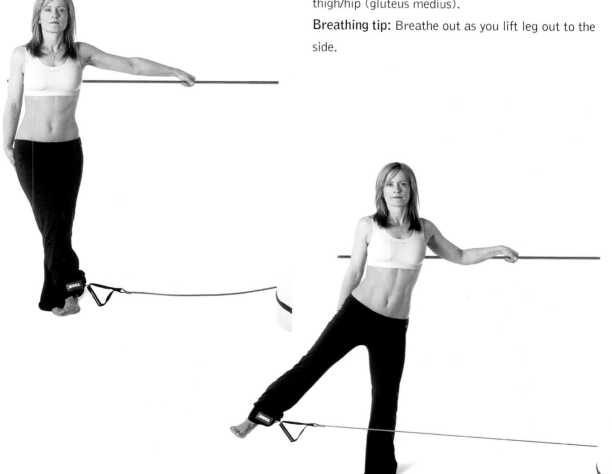

Inner Thigh

Sets: 2 / Repetitions: 12–15

Direction of resistance: From the closest side

Stand side-on to the anchor point. Attach one end of the band to an ankle strap, place it around the ankle of the leg that is closest to the anchor, and abduct (lift) your leg toward the anchor. You can place a stable object next to you to hold onto for support.

Whilst supporting your weight with one leg, draw the other across, bringing it in front of the supporting leg. Pause, and then bring it back across and out to the side, returning it to the start position. Repeat using your other leg. To make the exercise harder, step further away from the anchor point, or make it easier by moving closer.

Muscle group worked in this exercise: Inner thigh/hip (adductors).

Breathing tip: Breathe out as you bring your leg in.

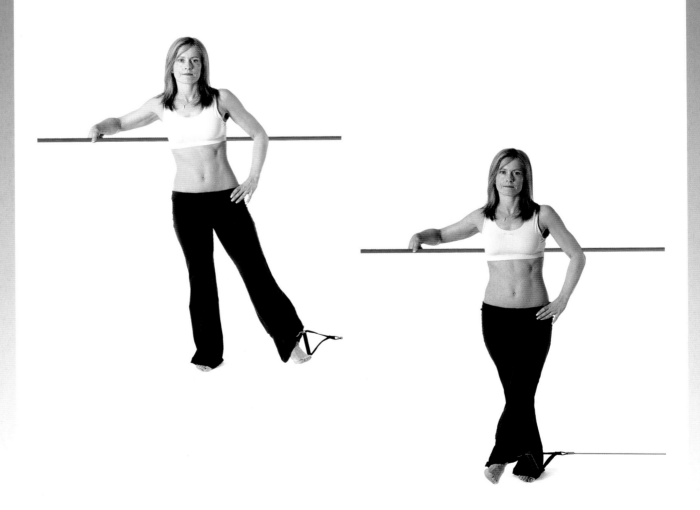

Standing Leg Extension

Sets: 2 / Repetitions: 12–15

Direction of resistance: From behind

Attach one end of the band to an ankle strap and then place the strap around the ankle of the leg you are starting on. With the band coming from behind you, stand on one leg, flexing the other at the hip so that the thigh is at 45 degrees. Bend the knee of the elevated leg so that your foot drops back. Place a stable object next to you to hold onto for support.

Extend your leg at the knee, keeping the upper part of the leg still, until your leg is straight. Pause, and then slowly bend the knee again, bringing your foot back to the starting position. Repeat using your other leg. To make the exercise harder, step further away from the anchor point, or you can make it easier by moving closer.

Muscle groups worked in this exercise: Front of thigh (quadriceps).

Breathing tip: Breathe out as you extend leg.

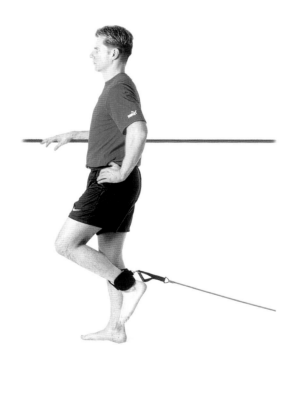

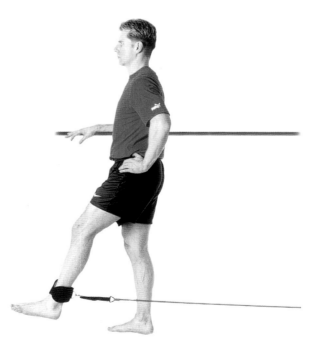

Calf Flex

Sets: 2 / Repetitions: 12–15

Direction of resistance: From above the foot

Place both resistance band handles around the ball of one foot. Take hold of the middle of the band with an overhand grip and bring hands up to chest level. Extend the leg with the band attached, so that it is straight and off the ground.

Push your toes down against the band, pivoting at the ankle, as if pushing on a brake pedal. Pause and then lift your toes back as far as possible, to the start position. Repeat with the other leg. You can move hands wider apart to make the exercise harder, or closer to make it easier.

Muscle group worked in this exercise: Back of lower leg (calf).

Breathing tip: Breathe out as you push toes down.

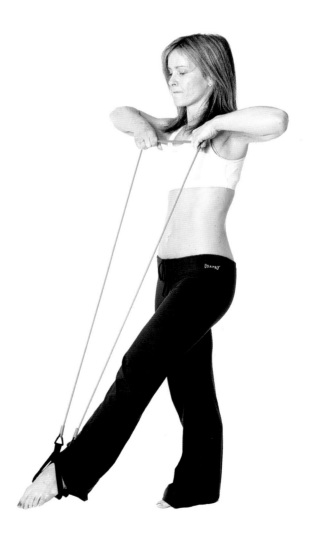

Abdominal Curl Twist

Sets: 2 / Repetitions: 12–15

Direction of resistance: No band required

Lie on your back, with your thighs at 90 degrees to your body and feet elevated to knee height. Touch fingertips to either side of your head. Breathe out and flatten your stomach as if pulling your belly button toward your lower back, then squeeze the muscles so that they are tight. Hold the contraction throughout the exercise.

   Lift and curl your shoulders toward your pelvis, rotating at the waist. Simultaneously flex your hip on the opposite side, bringing your knee toward the opposite elbow. Pause, and then slowly uncurl and extend the hip until you are back to the start position with both thighs level. Continue to repeat on the opposite side.

Muscle groups worked in this exercise: Center of abdomen (rectus abdominis), either side of abdomen (external obliques).

Breathing tip: Breathe out as you reach elbow to knee.

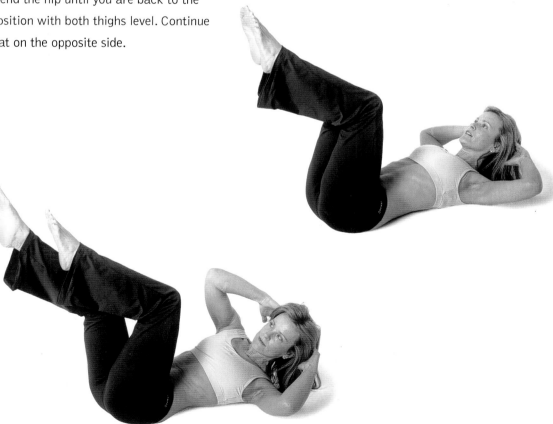

Abdominal Reverse Curl

Sets: 2 / Repetitions: 12–15

Direction of resistance: No band required

Lie flat on your back. Breathe out and flatten your stomach as if pulling your belly button toward your lower back then squeeze the muscles so that they are tight. Raise your legs so that your thighs are at 90 degrees to the floor and with feet elevated.

Raise your legs, bring your knees forward toward your head and push feet up. Your buttocks should lift from the floor very slightly. Pause, and then slowly uncurl, lowering your pelvis until your legs return to the start position. Focus on contracting your abdomen and not the movement of the legs. Keep your neck and shoulders relaxed and on the floor throughout the exercise.

Muscle groups worked in this exercise: Abdomen (rectus abdominis).

Breathing tip: Breathe out as you raise your legs toward you.

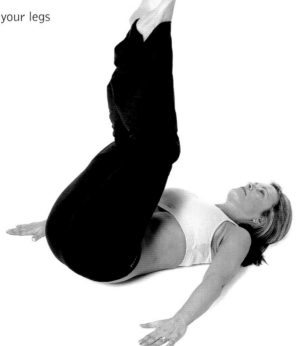

Dorsal Raises

Sets: 2 / Repetitions: 12–15

Direction of resistance: No band required

Lie flat on your front with head straight. Legs should also be straight and arms extended above your head.

Lift your left arm and right leg, extending it at the hip and keeping both arm and leg straight. Pause, and then slowly lower your arm and leg back down to the floor until you reach the start position. Then repeat with your right arm and left leg.

Muscle group worked in this exercise: Length of back (erector spinae).

Breathing tip: Breathe out as you lift opposite arm and leg.

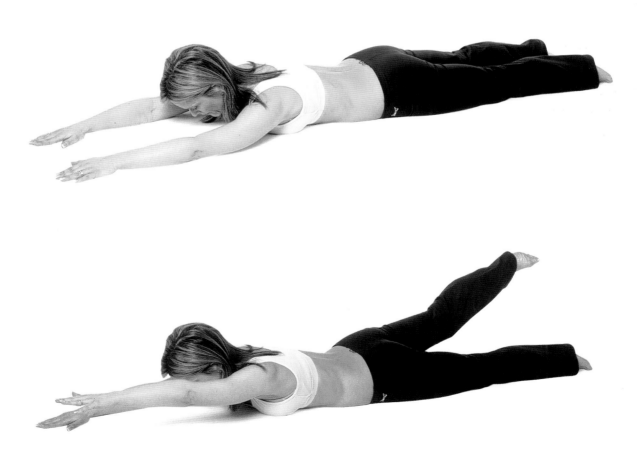

Resistance Band Golf Workout

Many top golfers are turning to resistance training to improve their fitness and game. It is important to train for sport, not only to enhance performance, but also to prevent injury by working the muscles around major joints for strength, power, and support.

Ensure that you warm up for at least 10 minutes before starting the workout (see page 72).

Lunge

Sets: 2 / Repetitions: 12–15

Direction of resistance: From under foot

From standing, take a large step forward with one foot and place the band underneath it. Keep both legs extended, feet parallel with your leading foot flat and the heel of your back foot raised. Hold the handles of the band with an overhand grip, and bring them up to shoulder level with the palms of your hands facing forward.

Bend your knees, stopping just before the knee of your back leg touches the floor, and both legs are bent to a 90-degree angle. Pause and then extend your legs, pushing through the heel of the leading leg until you are back to the start position. Try to keep your back as vertical as possible throughout the exercise. Ensure that the knee of your leading leg remains in line with your ankle as your knee bends.

Muscle groups worked in this exercise: Front of thigh (quadriceps), buttocks (gluteus maximus).
Breathing tip: Breathe out as you extend your legs.

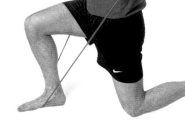

Hip Flexion

Sets: 2 / Repetitions: 12–15

Direction of resistance: From behind

Attach the band to an ankle strap then place it around the ankle of the leg that you are starting with. Position yourself so that the band is coming from behind you. Stand on one leg, extending the other at the hip and knee so that the thigh is at 30 degrees behind you. Keep your body upright and abdominal muscles tight. You can place a stable object next to you for support.

In a forward movement, flex your hip. Allow the knee to bend and lift knee as high as possible toward your chest without moving your back out of the upright position. Pause, and then slowly lower your knee, extending your hip and leg back to the starting position. Repeat using your other leg. Ensure that your upper body remains still throughout the exercise. To make the exercise harder, step further away from the anchor point, or make it easier by moving closer.

Muscle groups worked in this exercise: Hip flexors (iliopsoas).

Breathing tip: Breathe out as you lift knee.

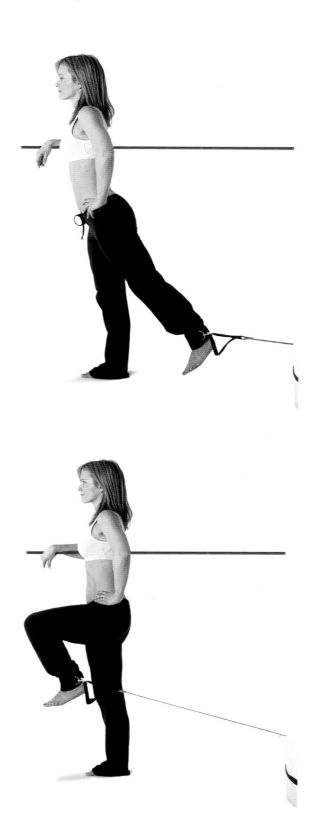

Standing Hamstring Curl

Sets: 2 / Repetitions: 12–15

Direction of resistance: From in front

Attach one end of the band to an ankle strap and then place around the ankle of the leg that you are starting with. You can place a stable object next to you to hold onto for support.

Flex one leg at the knee, until the lower leg is at 90 degrees to the upper. Pause, and then extend the leg at the knee until your leg is straight. Repeat using your other leg. Ensure that your hips remain still and keep both knees together throughout the exercise. To make the exercise harder, step further away from the anchor point, or make it easier by moving closer.

Muscle group worked in this exercise: Back of upper leg (hamstrings).

Breathing tip: Breathe out as you bend the knee.

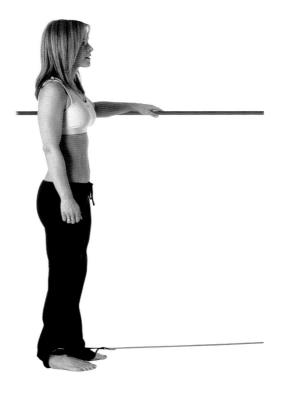
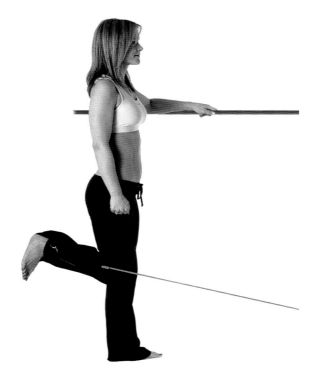

Calf Flex

Sets: 2 / Repetitions: 12–15

Direction of resistance: From above the foot

Place both resistance band handles around the ball of one foot. Take hold of the middle of the band with an overhand grip, and bring them up to chest level. Extend the leg with the band attached, so that it is straight and off the ground.

Push your toes down against the band, pivoting at the ankle, as if pushing on a brake pedal. Pause and then lift your toes back as far as possible, to the start position. Repeat with the other leg. You can move your hands wider apart to make the exercise harder, or closer to make it easier.

Muscle group worked in this exercise: Back of lower leg (calf).

Breathing tip: Breathe out as you push toes down.

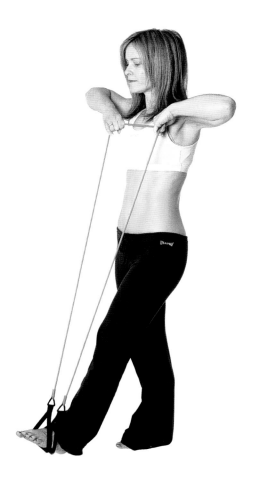
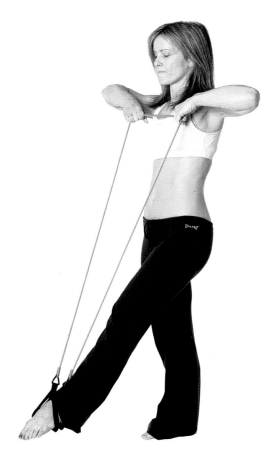

Close Grip Pull Down

Sets: 2 / Repetitions: 12–15

Direction of resistance: From above/in front

Kneel down facing the anchor point with the band coming from above you. Keep your back straight and abdominal muscles tight. Hold the handles with a close palms-in grip and arms extended toward the anchor point.

Pull the band down in a straight line by bending both arms, with elbows in tight, until your hands touch your chest. Pause, and then extend your arms following the same line, until they are back to the start position. Ensure that your back remains straight and still throughout the exercise to prevent any swaying back and forth.

Muscle groups worked in this exercise: Back (latissimus dorsi), back of shoulders (posterior deltoid), and front of upper arms (biceps).

Breathing tip: Breathe out as you pull down.

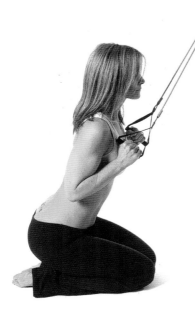

Upright Row

Sets: 2 / Repetitions: 12–15

Direction of resistance: From below

With the resistance band under the arches of both feet, place them hip-width apart. Swap the handles of the band to opposite hands so that it crosses over and hold them with a close overhand grip. Extend arms down toward the floor until they are straight, but don't round your shoulders.

With elbows leading, lift the handles of the band until your hands reach your chin, keeping them close to your body throughout the movement. Then return back to the start position, stopping when arms are fully extended. Ensure that your back remains still throughout the exercise. You can place feet wider apart to make the exercise harder, or closer to make it easier.

Muscle groups worked in this exercise: Upper back / neck (upper & lower trapezius), front and middle of shoulder (anterior & medial deltoid), and front of upper arms (biceps).

Breathing tip: Breathe out as you pull arms up.

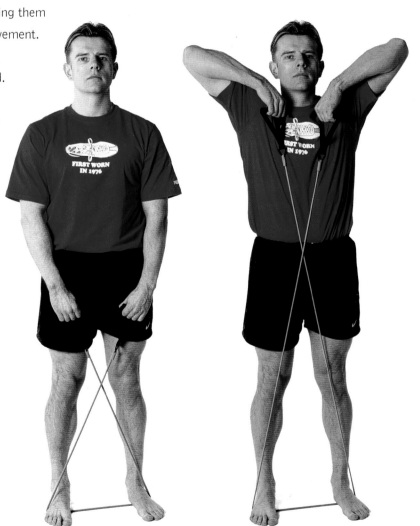

Chest Press

Sets: 2 / Repetitions: 12–15

Direction of resistance: From behind

Hold the handles of the band in each hand with an overhand grip and elbows bent at 90 degrees. Ensure that elbows and wrists are all elevated to shoulder height and are parallel to the floor.

Extend both arms forward until they are straight and then slowly bend arms back to the start position, stopping when you feel a slight stretch across your chest and shoulders. To make the exercise harder, step further forward, or make it easier by moving closer to the attachment.

Muscle groups worked in this exercise: Chest (pectorals), front of shoulders (anterior deltoid), and back of upper arms (triceps).

Breathing tip: Breathe out as you extend arms forward.

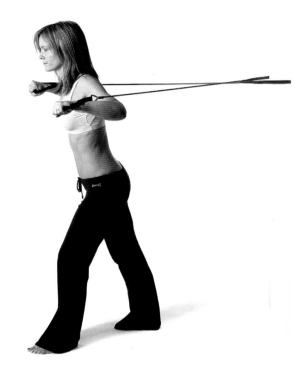

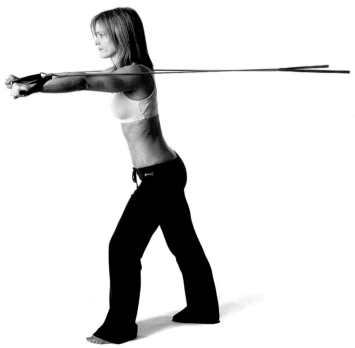

Shoulder Front Raise

Sets: 2 / Repetitions: 12–15

Direction of resistance: From below

Place the resistance band under the arches of both feet. Stand with feet hip-width apart, and in the correct standing exercise posture. Take hold of the handles with an overhand grip and arms straight by your side.

Lift your arms up in front of you, until your hands are just above shoulder height, pause, and then slowly bring arms back to the starting position, keeping arms extended throughout the full range of movement. Ensure that your back remains still throughout the exercise to prevent any swaying or throwing of weight. To make the exercise harder, keep feet further apart, or make it easier by moving them closer together.

Muscle group worked in this exercise: Front of shoulder (anterior deltoid).

Breathing tip: Breathe out as you bring your arms up.

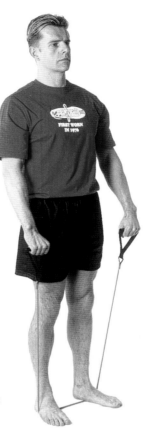

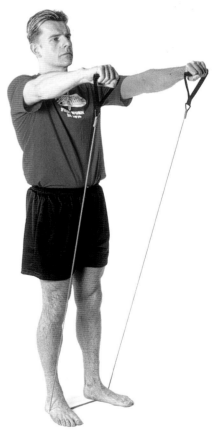

Reverse Flys

Sets: 2 / Repetitions: 12–15

Direction of resistance: From in front

Take hold of the handles with a palms-inward grip, your arms extended forward at shoulder height, and a very slight bend in the elbows. There should be tension in the band already.

Bring your arms apart and out to the side, keeping arms at shoulder height. Retract shoulder blades together, pause, and then slowly bring arms back to the starting position, with arms extended. Ensure that your back remains still throughout the exercise to prevent any swaying or loss of balance. To make the exercise harder, step further back, or make it easier by moving closer to the attachment.

Muscle groups worked in this exercise: Back of shoulder (posterior deltoid), between shoulder blades (rhomboids).

Breathing tip: Breathe out as you bring your arms out to the side.

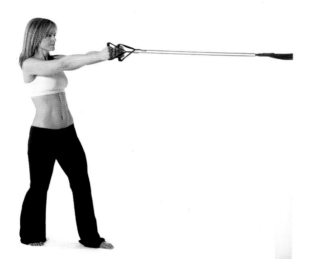

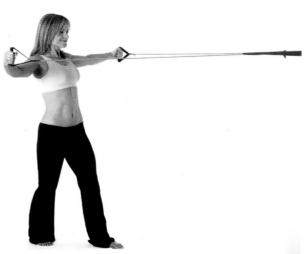

Bicep Hammer Curls

Sets: 2 / Repetitions: 12–15

Direction of resistance: From below

Place the resistance band under the arches of both feet. Stand with feet hip-width apart, and in the correct standing posture. Take hold of the handles with a palms-in grip and arms straight by your side.

Lift your hands in front of you by flexing at the elbow, keeping palms facing in and upper arms locked by your sides. Pause when your hands are at shoulder height and then slowly straighten arms back to the starting position, stopping when your hands reach the side of your legs. Ensure that your back and upper arms remain still throughout the exercise. To make the exercise harder, move feet further apart, or make it easier by moving them closer together.

Muscle group worked in this exercise: Front of upper arms (biceps).

Breathing tip: Breathe out as you bring your hands up.

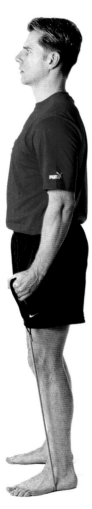
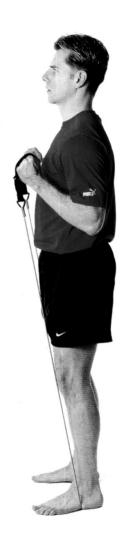

Triceps Kickbacks

Sets: 2 / Repetitions: 12–15

Direction of resistance: From in front

Stand with feet in a split stance, leaning upper body forward to about 45 degrees. Rest the hand that you're not using on the thigh of your leading leg for support. Take hold of one handle with a palm-in grip. Upper arm should remain close to your side, with elbow bent and elevated to shoulder height.

Extend your arm, pulling the handle back behind you until your arm is straight. Pause, and then bend your arm, returning your hand back to the start position. Keep your upper arm horizontal and held in position throughout the exercise. Repeat exercise with your other arm. To make the exercise harder, step further away from the anchor point or make it easier by moving closer.

Muscle group worked in this exercise: Back of upper arms (triceps).

Breathing tip: Breathe out as you extend arm back.

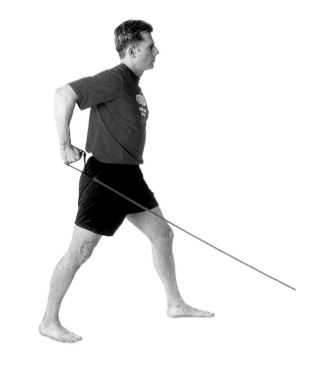

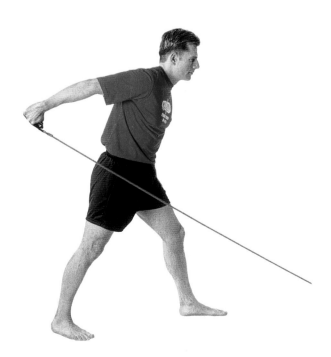

Standing External Shoulder Rotation

Sets: 2 / Repetitions: 12–15

Direction of resistance: From the opposite side

Stand in the correct exercise posture, sideways-on to the anchor point, with the band on the opposite side to the one that you're working. Hold one handle with a palm-in grip, bending arm 90 degrees at the elbow. Position your upper arm so that it is tight to your body. Get into the start position by rotating your shoulder so that your forearm is across your body.

Rotate your shoulder by swinging your forearm around to the side, pivoting your elbow on your hip, and stopping when it is parallel with the band. Pause, and then slowly allow your shoulder to rotate back by swinging your arm back across the front of your body, following the same line, until it reaches the start position.

Muscle groups worked in this exercise: Rotator cuff.
Breathing tip: Breathe out as you move your arm out to the side.

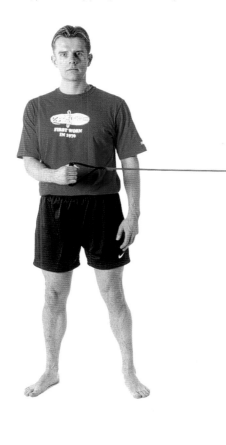
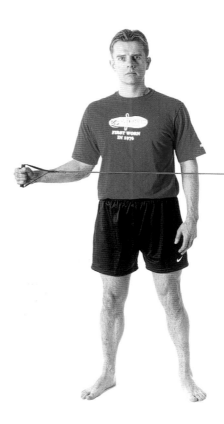

Lying Internal Shoulder Rotation

Sets: 2 / Repetitions: 12–15

Direction of resistance: From behind

Lie flat on your back so that the anchor point is above your head. Hold one handle with an underhand grip, bending arm at the elbow. Position your upper arm so that it is at a 90 degrees to your body with your shoulder and elbow touching the floor. Your hand should be at head level and as close to the floor as is comfortable.

Rotate your shoulder by lifting your hand up and over in an arc, pivoting on the elbow. Rotate your arm as far as is comfortable and without the shoulder lifting away from the floor. Pause, and then slowly allow your shoulder to rotate back by lifting your hand back up and over following the same line, until it is back to the start position.

Muscle groups worked in this exercise: Rotator cuff.
Breathing tip: Breathe out as you move your hand in the direction of your feet.

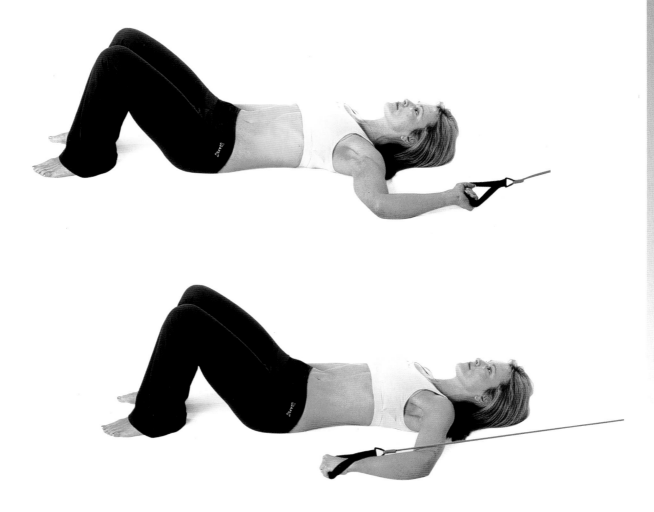

Abdominal Curl Twist

Sets: 2 / Repetitions: 12–15

Direction of resistance: No band required

Lie on your back, with your thighs at 90 degrees to your body and feet elevated to knee height. Touch fingertips to either side of your head. Breathe out and flatten your stomach as if pulling your belly button toward your lower back then squeeze the muscles so that they are tight. Hold the contraction throughout the exercise.

Lift and curl your shoulders toward your pelvis, rotating at the waist. Simultaneously flex your hip on the opposite side, bringing your knee toward the opposite elbow. Pause, and then slowly uncurl and extend the hip until you are back to the start position with both thighs level. Continue and repeat on the opposite side.

Muscle groups worked in this exercise: Center of abdomen (rectus abdominis), either side of abdomen (external obliques).

Breathing tip: Breathe out as you reach your elbow to knee.

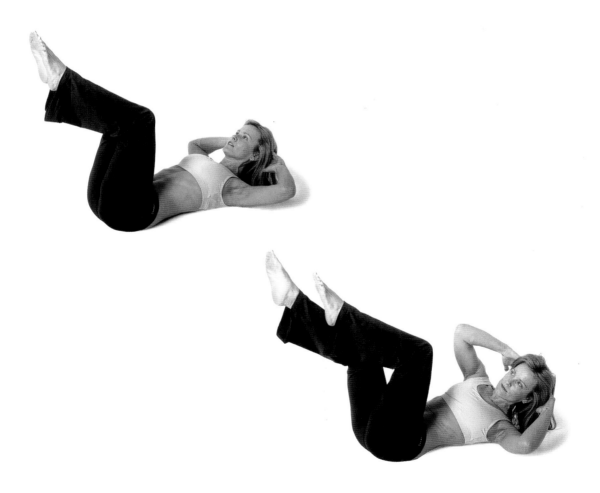

Dorsal Raises

Sets: 2 / Repetitions: 12–15

Direction of resistance: No band required

Lie flat on your front with head straight. Legs should also be straight and arms extended above your head.

Lift your left your arm and right leg, extending it at the hip, and keeping both arm and leg straight. Pause, and then slowly lower your arm and leg back down to the floor until you reach the start position. Then repeat with your right arm and left leg.

Muscle group worked in this exercise: Length of back (erector spinae).

Breathing tip: Breathe out as you lift opposite arm and leg.

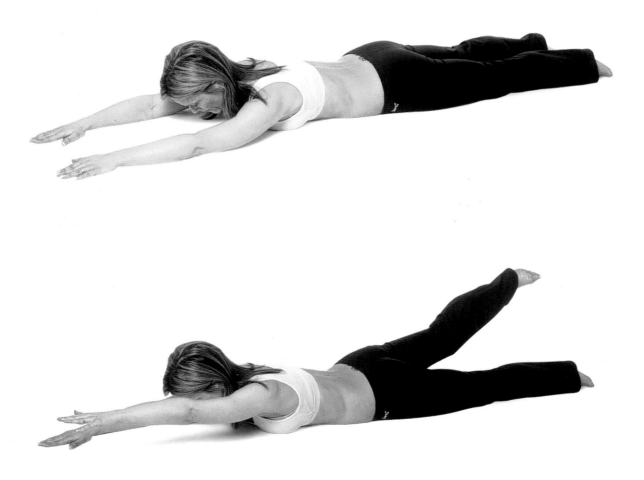

Index